Summer
fit

igloobooks

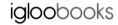

Published in 2016
by Igloo Books Ltd
Cottage Farm
Sywell
NN6 0BJ
www.igloobooks.com

Cover images © iStock / Getty

LEO002 0316
2 4 6 8 10 9 7 5 3 1
ISBN: 978-1-78557-342-2

Cover designed by Charles Wood-Penn
Designed by Charles Wood-Penn
Edited by Natalie Baker

Printed and manufactured in China

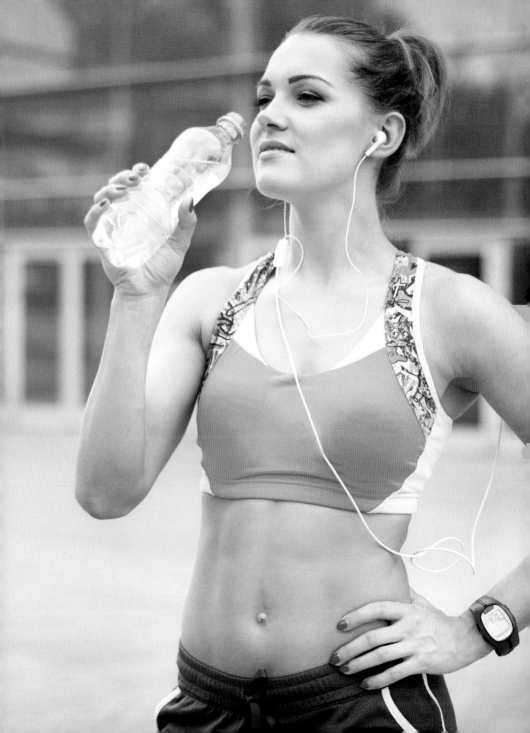

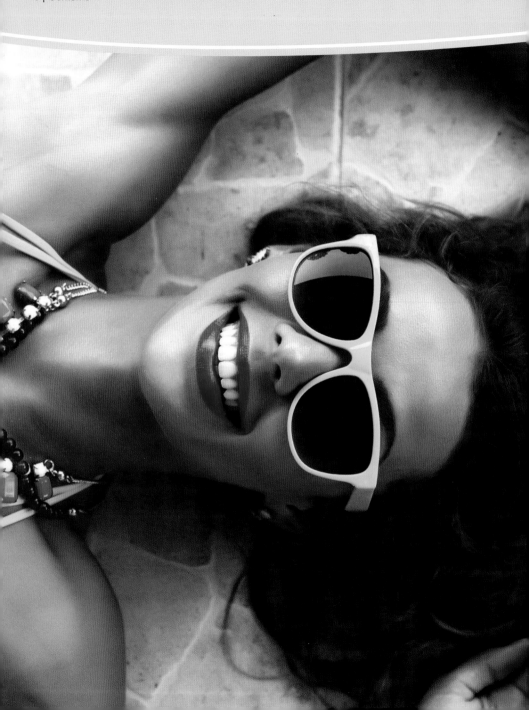

Contents

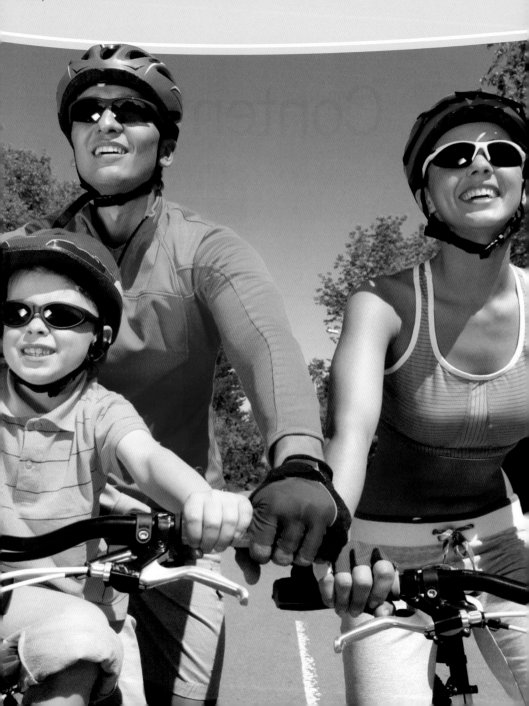

Introduction

As the days get longer and the scent of summer begins to lift our spirits, thoughts turn to feeling and looking good for the holidays. It is easy to sink into a winter lifestyle of comfort food and curling up under a blanket on dark nights. We then emerge like a sleepy animal, blinking, stretching and feeling groggy and tired. But don't be disheartened, the great outdoors is waiting for you to shed your winter coat and get active once again!

What is summer fitness?

Summer fitness means different things to different people. Many of us want to look good, with toned arms and slender legs to show off in our shorts and vests. Seasonal eating also brings an enticing array of salads and fresh produce, encouraging us to eat our way to a healthier, fitter body.

Lifestyle changes

Getting into shape for summer means making a change from your winter habits. Seize the sunshine ethos and embark upon a routine of exercise and healthy eating that will challenge and strengthen your body, increase your energy levels and allow you to embrace the months ahead. Get ready to feel great!

Goal Getters

The key to success is to pinpoint exactly what you want to achieve. Make a list of your targets and break them down into a plan of action. Do your summer clothes feel tighter than they did last year? Do you feel sluggish and wish you had more energy? Do you want to get active again?

Once you have written down your objectives, consider them in both the short term and the long term. Don't expect miracles: this is YOUR project and YOU are going to have to work to see results.

Don't diet

It sounds too good to be true, but it is well documented that people who follow diets struggle to maintain their weight loss. In the short term, your aim should be to eat better, which is not necessarily the same as eating less. Substitute bad foods for good (see pages 12–17 for advice on how to do this). Your long-term goal could be to remain 10 pounds lighter than you are today, while still providing your body with the healthy fuel it needs.

Get fitter

The fittest people are not necessarily those who look the best in their beach wear. The friend who can run a marathon may still complain that her bottom looks large in a pair of jeans. The guy who can outpace you on the rowing machine is carrying a few extra pounds on his waistline. However, they know their body and have trained it and nurtured it to get the best performance from it. In the short term, focus on upping your cardiovascular exercise. In the long term, look to maintain your desired level of fitness without getting bored of your exercise regime.

Look great!

An increase in cardio exercise will lift your spirits and help you burn calories. It will begin to tone your muscles and reduce body fat. However, if your short-term goal is to look better in a bikini, you should include targeted muscle toning in your regime. By varying the exercises you do, you will reap long-term improvements in bone density and core strength, which will improve your posture and body image, and help to prevent injuries and back pain.

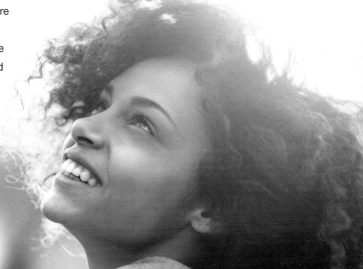

Time for a Change

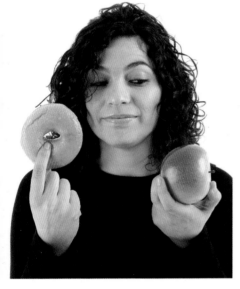

It doesn't take a genius to work out that if you don't make changes in your habits, your body won't change – at least, not for the better. Exercise and healthy eating go hand in hand, and you should anticipate tackling both of them together.

However, don't try to change everything all at once. Your body won't know what's hit it! Assess your eating habits and make small changes. Eat more veg and drink less wine, or cut out second helpings. Concentrate on the good things and don't get too worried if you slip back to being 'bad' from time to time.

Fighting fit

Focus on your exercise regime. Think about things that have failed you before and figure out what went wrong. Maybe you're looking to kickstart a regime that has worked until now but has reached a stalemate, with a plateau in your weight loss or fitness levels. Answer these three questions to get yourself on track:

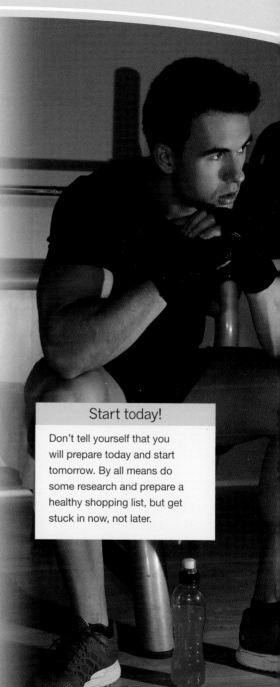

Why do you want to change?

Be clear about your goal. Are you worried about how you'll look by the pool or how many lengths of it you can swim? Do you want to wear shorts instead of covering up with cropped trousers? A strong mental image will help you make the right choices.

How will you change?

What new habits are you going to form that will get you into shape? A vague promise to 'do some exercise' isn't enough. If you have joined a gym, when exactly are you going to go, and what are you going to do with your time there? If you don't like the gym, what will you do instead?

Who will help?

Enlist help from friends with similar goals. Tell people what you are doing and ask them to encourage you rather than entice you back into bad habits.

Start today!

Don't tell yourself that you will prepare today and start tomorrow. By all means do some research and prepare a healthy shopping list, but get stuck in now, not later.

Eat Fit

Regular exercise is crucial if you want to maintain a healthy body, but you will struggle to lose weight or inches if you don't watch what you eat. In fact, as you increase your energy output, you may need more food than before.

Don't start your summer fitness campaign thinking that you have to go hungry. All too often, people are afraid of food. It is portrayed as the enemy of weight loss, and sometimes it can be, but you can graze all day long if you eat properly.

The right stuff

Look at exactly what you eat. How much of it do you love? What could you manage without? It's surprising how habits dictate what we consume. Keep a food diary for a week and then review it. Do you finish lunch each day with a biscuit that you barely even notice? Do you eat yogurt as dessert and not even enjoy it? Take them out of your diet for a few days and see if you truly miss them. If you're hungry an hour after lunch, snack on healthy fillers instead, such as fruit, nuts or a sliver of cheese.

Getting smaller

Doing exercise on a full stomach will take its toll, so aim to eat small amounts at more regular intervals. Serve yourself a smaller portion and don't eat a single mouthful more if you feel full. You can still eat your favourite treats, but cut them in half. Remember that a treat is something you allow yourself once in a while. If you have the willpower to exercise regularly, you also have the willpower to say no to foods that are counter productive.

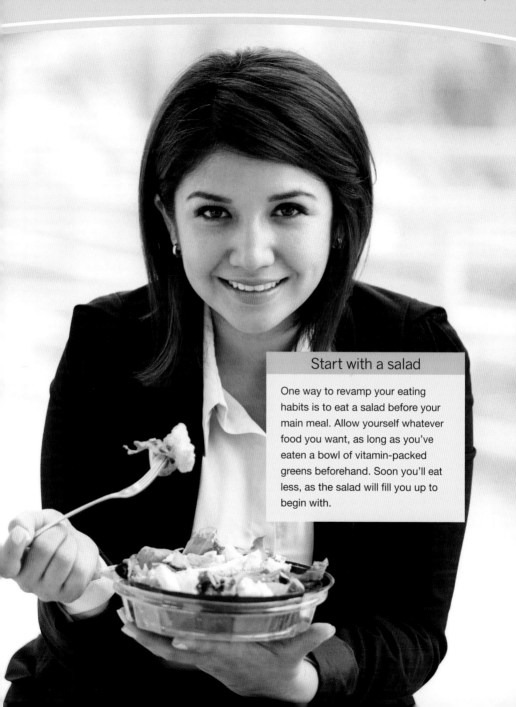

Start with a salad

One way to revamp your eating habits is to eat a salad before your main meal. Allow yourself whatever food you want, as long as you've eaten a bowl of vitamin-packed greens beforehand. Soon you'll eat less, as the salad will fill you up to begin with.

Fully fuelled

The market is overloaded with drinks and food supplements that claim to improve sporting performance. Be wary. You probably don't need them. Anyone undertaking less than an hour of exercise per session can get their fuel from everyday foods.

Despite their bad press, carbs can be your fitness friend. They are the main source of energy during exercise and keep your brain working and your heart pumping. Become carb-savvy; simple carbs such as fruit will give you an instant energy boost to get you started. Complex carbs, such as wholegrains and high-fibre cereal, are digested more slowly and will provide your body with a steady release of energy.

Food for thought

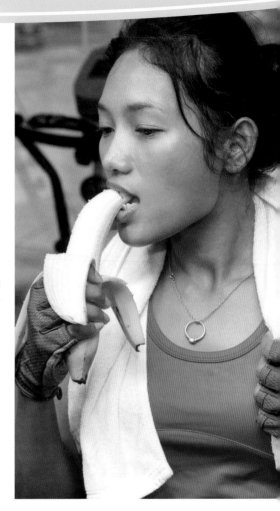

A moderately active person (you!) should aim for a diet made up of around 60 per cent carbs, 20 per cent fat and 20 per cent protein. Cut out refined grains found in crackers, cakes and white varieties of pasta, bread and rice. Instead, get your carbs from fibre-rich vegetables and pulses, which are naturally lower in calories as well. Try yogurt and nuts for a great start to the day, or fruit and a slice of wholemeal toast. Eat a light snack about an hour before your workout.

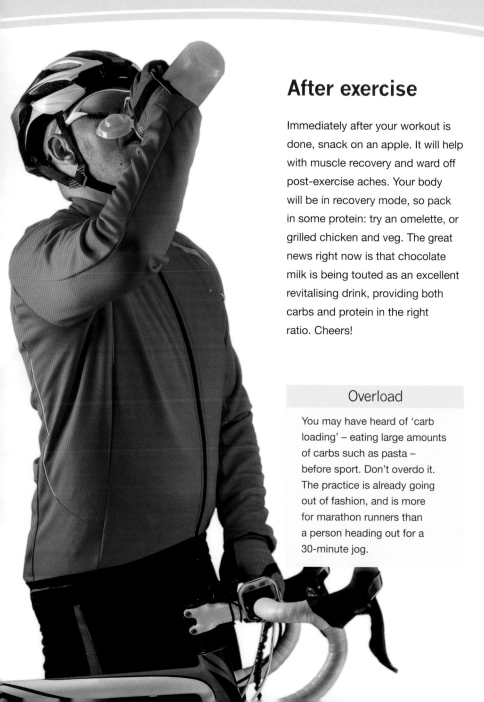

After exercise

Immediately after your workout is done, snack on an apple. It will help with muscle recovery and ward off post-exercise aches. Your body will be in recovery mode, so pack in some protein: try an omelette, or grilled chicken and veg. The great news right now is that chocolate milk is being touted as an excellent revitalising drink, providing both carbs and protein in the right ratio. Cheers!

Overload

You may have heard of 'carb loading' – eating large amounts of carbs such as pasta – before sport. Don't overdo it. The practice is already going out of fashion, and is more for marathon runners than a person heading out for a 30-minute jog.

Ditch it!

There is so much in the media about food that it's hard not to know the basics of everyday eating. It's all pretty simple stuff. Here are some simple no-go items that should ring warning bells.

- **Cakes and biscuits**: whilst there may be hidden sugar in baked beans and ketchup, there is a lot more sugar that's plain to see and easy to limit. A tough workout can use around 500 calories an hour. However, a single shortbread finger is 90 calories, a jam doughnut is 250 calories and a large chocolate muffin is 500 calories. Is it worth it?

- **Ready meals**: microwave meals often provide less nutrition than homemade versions. A 430 gram spaghetti bolognese ready meal typically provides more than one-third of your daily recommended amount of salt and fat but very few minerals and vitamins. If you make your own you can limit the salt content, drain off excess fat and load it with vegetables.

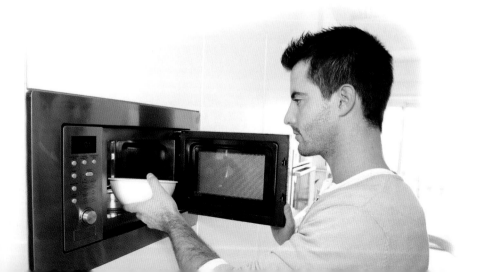

- **Fizzy drinks**: to rehydrate, drink water. To socialize with friends, have a coffee. Treat yourself with an occasional glass of wine, if that's your reward after a hard day. But stay away from sugary drinks. Cola and other fizzy drinks contain chemicals that may leach minerals from your bones, and many flavoured waters are full of sugar.

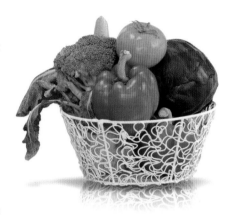

- **Grab bags**: if you want to lose weight, don't buy in bulk. It is difficult to estimate a healthy portion from a large bag and you will inevitably eat more than you intended.

What should you eat?

Use plant-based foods as your staple items and make sure you provide enough fuel for your lifestyle.

- **Protein**: look for low-calorie, high protein foods, such as tuna, salmon, eggs, cheese, yogurt, beans and pulses.

- **Fats**: good fats ease joints and regulate your heart rhythm. They include avocado, hummus, seeds and nuts, and veggies roasted in olive oil.

- **Fresh produce**: aim to 'eat a rainbow' throughout the week, made up of fresh fruit and vegetables. Go heavy on the greens and purples, with fewer whites and yellows. Excellent examples are leafy greens (spinach, kale, cabbage) and purple or red berries. Not only will they provide vitamins and antioxidants, but they are also an excellent source of fibre. You need around 14 grams of fibre for every 1,000 calories you consume.

Mindset Matters

Getting into shape is all about getting into your groove. Your aim is to change your habits in such a way that exercising regularly and eating well becomes a way of life.

Schedule it in

Create an exercise routine that suits your lifestyle. Most people find it easiest to get their run or swim out of the way first thing. Prepare any clothes or exercise gear the night before and set your alarm so you can simply get up and go. Don't wait for motivation to hit you; it might not! Simply accept that you're working out tomorrow because it's Wednesday and that's what you do. If mornings don't suit your timetable, find a time that does. Maybe you have an hour in the evening when your daughter is at dance class, or a long lunch on Friday when everyone else goes to the pub? Don't be swayed by a busy schedule – set aside your exercise time in the same way that you would plan a meeting, and stick to it.

Go public

Tell people what you are doing – announce it on social media, inform your family and friends, let your colleagues know why you disappear three lunchtimes a week. Not only will it allow them to support and encourage you, it will motivate you to not give up. Who wants to be seen to fall short of their targets?

A social side

Join forces with someone who has the same goals as you. You can encourage and educate each other, and if you're the competitive type, you will drive each other on. Don't be afraid that your new routine will cancel out your social life; simply shift your socializing to fit your workouts. Persuade the friends you meet for coffee to go for a walk instead. You can still chat, but you're less likely to eat cake!

Teamwork

The other bonus to finding an exercise buddy is the motivation you can offer one another. Leaving the house to run in the rain might not be appealing, but if you know your friend will be waiting for you, you won't want to let her down. Your bad days will be her good days, and you will push each other when you just don't have your own personal drive.

Diary dates

If your target is to look good on holiday, mark the date in bold in your calendar. Add other events that might put obstacles in your way – a birthday party or a weekend with friends – so you can work around them.

Quantity and Quality

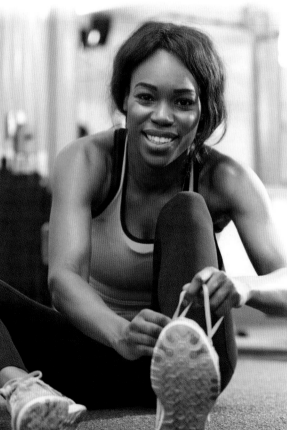

How much exercise should you aim for and how often should you be doing it? The recommended level for healthy adults is 150 minutes per week, split into three or four sessions with rest days in between. If you need to exercise two days in a row to fit into your schedule, let your body guide you. Don't overdo it and burn yourself out, but go for it if you feel strong and energized. Try different disciplines or target different parts of your body on consecutive days.

Get moving!

Be honest with yourself; have you done nothing all day when you know you really should? Get off the sofa and lunge around the room. It will kickstart you into moving more.

Cardio, strength and flexibility

For a fully toned, healthy body, you should aim to vary your exercise. There are three basic workout types. Cardio, or endurance training, will increase your stamina and help your heart. Cycling, running, swimming and using gym equipment such as the cross trainer and rowing machine all give you a cardio workout. Strength exercises build muscle tone. This needn't be lifting weights; floor work such as squats and lunges also count. Flexibility exercises such as yoga, Pilates and tai chi help to shape and stretch your muscles and joints. They also strengthen your core muscles which will improve your posture and body image, and help to prevent back problems.

Super sports

Don't worry if you're not a fan of running or the gym. Many activities offer a good all-round workout and can be great fun. Boxing, dancing, skiing, surfing and rowing all raise your heart rate and work a variety of muscle groups. A 60-minute game of squash typically burns more than 800 calories for someone who weighs 11 stone. It also ticks the boxes for lunging, jumping, sprinting and twisting, works the upper and lower body, and raises your heart rate. All the same things you would incorporate into a gym session, with the added bonuses of improved balance, agility, co-ordination and stress-busting.

Aerobic and anaerobic

Many types of exercise are aerobic. They increase and improve your body's oxygen consumption. Generally, cardio workouts and any activity done at a steady pace with a moderate intensity level are aerobic. Anaerobic exercise builds muscle mass and increases power. Strength exercises, whether done with equipment or using your own body weight as resistance, are anaerobic.

Sports Science

As you delve into the world of fitness and weight loss, you will come across certain concepts and terms that are regularly used.

Body Mass Index

Your Body Mass Index, or BMI, is a number that determines whether you fall within an accepted weight for your height. If it is too high, you are carrying more weight than is healthy. The scale is skewed slightly if you are exceptionally tall or muscular, but on the whole it is a good general guide to what your target weight should be. There are several BMI calculators online.

Metabolic rate

This is the speed at which chemical reactions in your body allow cells to release energy from food. It indicates how many calories you burn at rest (basal metabolic rate) and during physical activity. It increases as you exercise and stays high for a while afterwards. As you become fitter, your basal metabolic rate increases, so you burn more calories even when you are not active. Double bonus!

Give yourself a boost

Spicy foods such as chilli and curry are thought to raise your metabolism by as much as 50 per cent for two or three hours after you eat. Green tea also has a boosting effect, as does being hot or cold. So take a sauna or an icy dip!

Muscle map

As you read through the exercises later in this book, you will learn how to target different areas of your body for toning and strengthening muscles. This will give you a firmer, leaner body shape. Familiarize yourself with these muscles and you will be more aware of how to tackle problem areas such as your waist, bottom or thighs. Some areas, however, don't contain muscles, and losing inches will simply require weight loss.

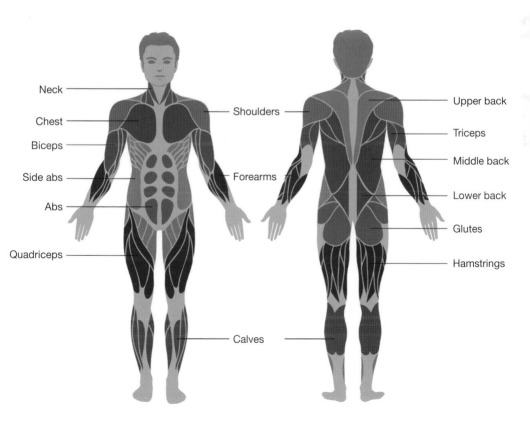

Neck

Chest

Biceps

Side abs

Abs

Quadriceps

Shoulders

Forearms

Calves

Upper back

Triceps

Middle back

Lower back

Glutes

Hamstrings

Beat the Boredom

Many people hurl themselves at a summer fitness campaign, work like crazy, then stop after only a few weeks. Two of the main obstacles are a plateau in visible results and sheer boredom. Be prepared for this, and shake things up in times of trouble.

Change

If your weight loss has stopped, or your fitness levels are no longer improving, it's time for a change. Your body is remarkable in many ways, but one characteristic of the human body is that it quickly adapts. What was a shock four weeks ago has now become the new normal. Keep your body on its toes and throw something new at it! Switch gym classes and try boxercise, or lose one running session and go for a swim. As summer arrives, head outdoors and play with the kids, or look for an outdoor gym or trim trail. Research shows that exercising in the open air boosts both physical and mental health compared with being inside.

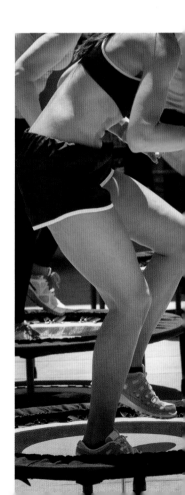

Do more

You might feel that you're already devoting several hours to exercise that could easily be spent doing something else, but don't panic! You don't need to leave the ironing unironed so you can spend more time in the pool. However, you can multitask. Do butt squeezes while you wait for the iron to heat up, or lunges as you empty the dishwasher. Even sitting with your legs or arms aloft from time to time while you watch TV will get your muscles in shape.

Have fun!

If exercise has become boring, then liven it up. Look online for clubs that offer more unusual activities or lessons such as rock climbing, fencing, pole dancing or horseriding. Try skipping or hulahooping, or play dodgeball or rounders in a group. Think outside the box; there are many kids' play areas that now offer fitness classes on their trampolines and climbing walls.

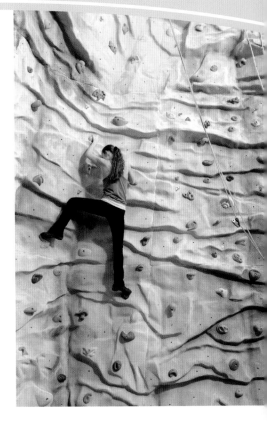

Turn on the TV

Invest in an exercise DVD to try something you haven't done before. There are literally thousands now available and many offer unusual exercise that may not be available to you locally. Search for zumbastep, ugi, animal flow, pound drumming workouts, groove, bokwa, katami or ropes gone wild, to name but a few!

Cut it Out

We all have our weak spots, but what exactly is your vice doing to your body as you wallow in a post-workout glow? You'd be surprised.

Drinking alcohol

Personal trainers usually recommend that you avoid alcohol on the same day as a workout. Alcohol restricts muscle recovery and slows muscle growth.

Sore head, sore muscles

Alcohol can increase inflammation in the muscles, so drinking after a tough training session can make you feel more sore than you otherwise would and increase your recovery time.

Alcohol dehydrates you when your body really needs extra hydration to replace lost fluids. It places additional stress on your liver and uses up vital amino acids that would otherwise be employed in fighting those nasty free radicals we hear so much about. Beer, wine and spirits (and the mixers that you put with them) are laden with calories without providing any nutrition.

Free radicals

These are groups of highly reactive atoms that can trigger chain reactions in the body, leading to the breakdown of cells. They are linked to skin ageing and cancer. Extreme endurance exercise can generate a higher than normal level of free radicals because of the increased use of oxygen in our cells. However, regular low-level exercise can enhance our antioxidant defences. Antioxidants are nature's warriors; they stabilize the atoms and prevent cell damage. They are found in all plant-based foods and in larger doses in orange produce (carrots, sweet potatoes, pumpkin) and foods that are high in Vitamin C.

Smoking

The dangers of smoking are widely known, but what if you light up straight after exercise? Once you have stretched and cooled down, your body uses extra oxygen to help your heart and muscles recover. Smoking replaces some of the body's oxygen with carbon dioxide. This reduces the oxygen available to the brain, which can add to any feeling of fatigue or even lightheadedness you might experience after exercise. Smoke inhalation narrows your airways and makes it harder to take in as much air as your body requires for recovery. Regular smoking also puts extra pressure on your heart and lungs.

Smoking sends billions of free radicals racing through your body. They attack tissue, causing lung disease and skin deterioration. Recent studies suggest that e-cigarettes also produce large amounts of free radicals.

Getting Started

So, your targets are set, your goals are visualized, your cupboards and body are fully stocked with healthy food. The next step is the big one: actually exercising. Of course, you can't step out in jeans and flip flops – you will need to be prepared. Here's a quick checklist before you break into a sweat.

Equipment

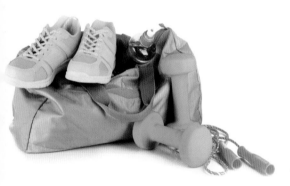

Most exercise requires very little equipment. If you're a lapsed athlete you may already have trainers, a water bottle and some form of sports clothing. For yoga or Pilates you will need looser clothing and a mat. Women should make sure they wear a suitable sports bra.

Money matters

If you're new to all this, don't go out and buy expensive items. Many sports shops will watch you run on a treadmill to assess your gait and offer advice on the best trainers for you. Don't be persuaded that expensive is better, but do listen to their advice on how you run and choose footwear accordingly. Likewise, most gyms offer a free trial session in the hope that you will sign up for membership. Do the rounds of all your local ones – you will benefit from cost-free exercise for a while and be able to decide which suits your needs the best.

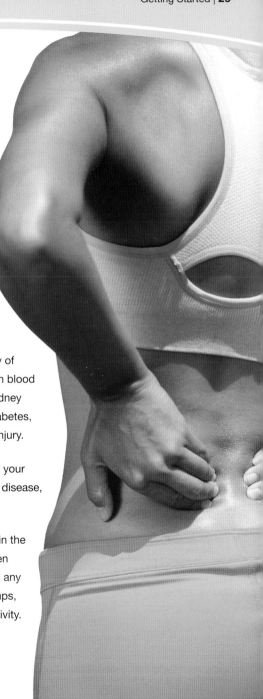

Sporting life

Of course, many sports do require more specialist items. However, if you're unsure what your regime will involve, consider borrowing a racquet or even a bike before you invest.

Health check

There are some important health issues to consider before you embark on your fitness campaign.

If you have ever been diagnosed with any of the following, seek a doctor's advice: high blood pressure or cholesterol, any heart/liver/kidney conditions, asthma, epilepsy, arthritis, diabetes, hernia or any recent or severe muscular injury.

Consult a health professional if anyone in your immediate family has suffered from heart disease, stroke or raised cholesterol.

Seek advice if you have been in hospital in the last 12 months, are pregnant or have given birth in the last year, or have experienced any chest pain, muscular pain, swelling, cramps, dizziness or fainting during strenuous activity.

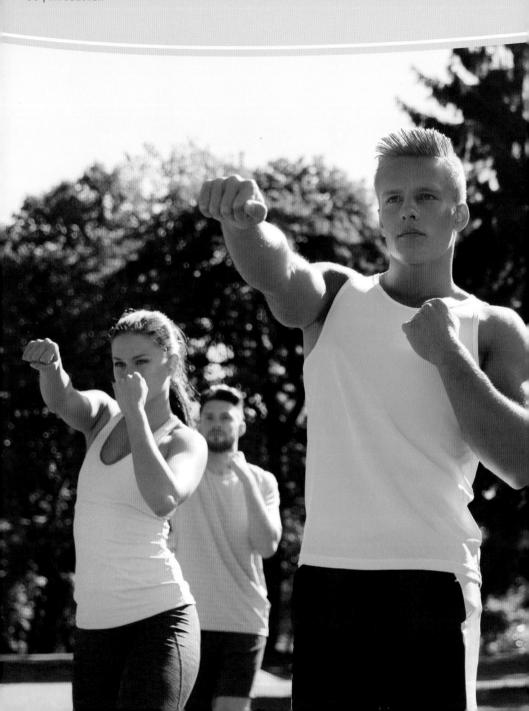

Active Fit

Choosing a broad range of activities will get you fit faster, and shape and tone your body in different places. Mix it up with cardio, such as running, cycling or swimming, and any sports-based activities that you enjoy, and a selection of power moves and stretches. Each of the following sections will tell you about the benefits and techniques for a selection of moves and activities, to ensure that you target problem areas and get a workout that suits your individual needs.

Body building

Don't be scared to use weights as part of your training. Keep the weights fairly light and you will build strength rather than bulk.

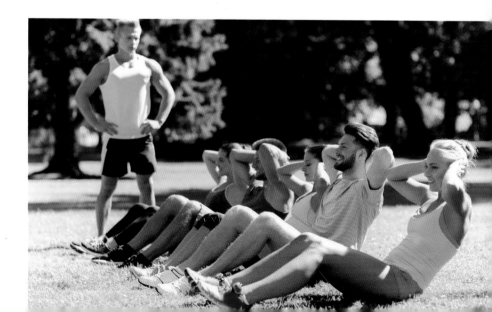

All the Right Moves

If you think that gym workouts are boring and repetitive, think again. There are so many different moves that you can include in your workout. There are certain classics, however, that really hit the target and never go out of fashion. Try to incorporate these basic moves into your weekly workouts: pushing, pulling and squatting.

Pushing or pressing against a weight with your arms works your shoulders, chest and triceps. Pulling, such as upright rows or chin-ups, shapes your forearms and biceps and strengthens your rear delts and back. Squats target your major leg muscles and your glutes. Each of these three types of move will help with balance and stability through your core and abs.

Excellent exercises

A personal training routine should see you lifting, dipping, crunching and jumping, but ensure that you cover the tried and tested 'big five': press-ups, planks, lunges, squats and pull-ups. Each of these, and variations of them, is dealt with on the following pages.

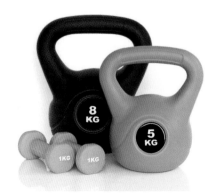

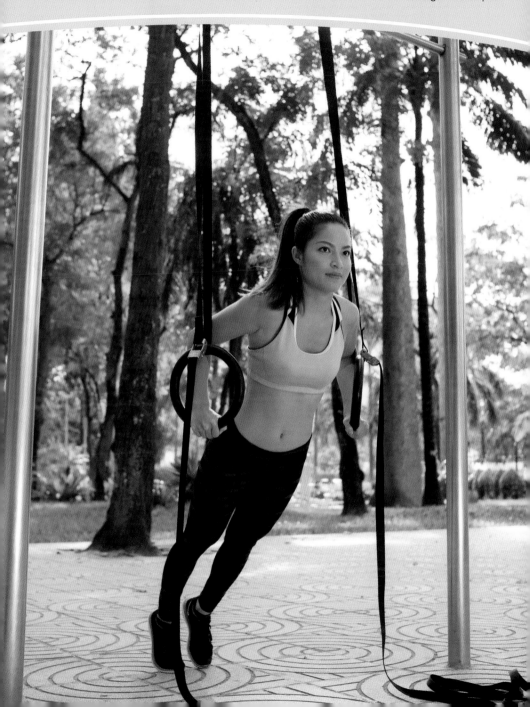

Floor Work: Abs and Core

Getting a flat stomach isn't only about your abs. There are several muscle groups that shape your midriff. Your aim is to work both upper and lower abs, obliques, tranverse abdominis and your lower back. Not only will you strengthen your core muscles, you will improve your posture and help to prevent back pain.

When working your middle section, be aware of what's going on inside you. Keep your muscles engaged for each movement, focusing on keeping your spine in a 'neutral' position with your pelvis neither tipped forwards nor backwards. Be careful not to jerk or strain your neck when doing sit-up movements. Let your hands support your head rather than pulling on it. Or you could rest your fingertips lightly behind your ears.

Do the following exercises in sets of three for 10 repetitions (reps) each, or for five minutes. Then move on to another part of your body.

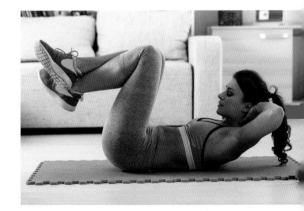

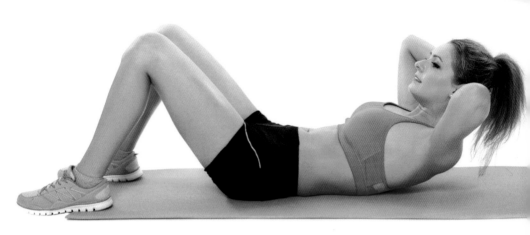

Crunches

Simple crunches will help to flatten your stomach. Learn to perform them properly to avoid straining your spine. Support your head, rest your fingers lightly behind your ears or keep your arms crossed over your chest. Alternatively, place your arms alongside you with your hands outstretched on the floor.

Relax!

To prevent yourself tensing the wrong muscles while you perform crunches, raise your tongue to the roof of your mouth.

To begin, lie on your back on a mat or carpet. Bend your knees and keep your feet flat on the floor, shoulder-width apart. Gaze at the ceiling and slowly raise your shoulders and chest. Do not lift your whole back off the floor, or tuck your chin into your chest. Hold this position for a second, looking between your knees, and engage your stomach muscles. Lower yourself back to the ground.

Focus on your breathing. For crunches and other exercises, breathe in through your nose and out through your mouth. Inhale at the start and exhale during the crunch. Inhale again as you release the move.

Sit-ups

This exercise is so easy to do, no matter where you are. You can even do it in a hotel room, so no excuses for skipping your summer fit workout! Sit-ups help strengthen and develop your stomach muscles and also work your hips and quads.

Lie on your back with your knees bent and feet planted flat on the floor. Your arms should be in one of the same positions as for crunches (see page 35).

Squeeze your shoulders back as though you are trying to pull your shoulder blades closer together. Tighten your abs and curl up, raising your chest to your bent knees. Tip your chin upwards slightly to maintain a good position. Exhale as you sit up. Hold for a second then inhale as you lower your body back to the floor in a controlled way.

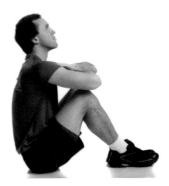

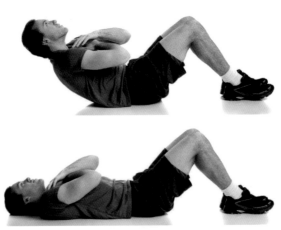

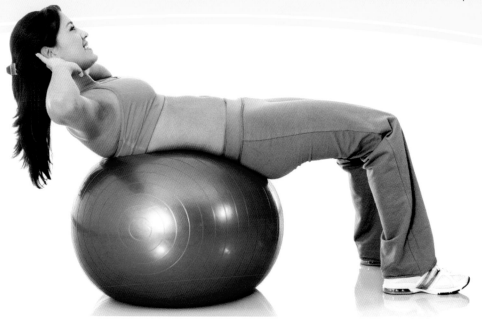

Crunches on an exercise ball

Working out with an exercise ball has a double benefit. The soft surface puts less pressure on your back than working out on the floor. It also uses your core muscles to help keep you stable.

Sit on the ball and place your hands behind your ears. Walk your feet forwards so that your upper body rolls back onto the ball. The ball should support your lower back. Ensure that your knees form at least a right angle.

Exhale and lift your upper body about 45 degrees. Pull in your abs from the belly button. Breathe in and lower your body back to the starting position. Don't use your hands to pull your head or neck, but focus on the muscles in your stomach. Try to keep your elbows pointed out to the side, not forwards.

Proper posture

To position your chin properly, imagine you have an orange tucked underneath it.

Russian twists

Here's another exercise that's great to do any time, anywhere. It not only works your central abs but targets the oblique muscles that define your waist.

Sit on the floor with your knees bent and your heels resting on the ground. Lean slightly back and hold your arms outstretched in front of you. Your fingers should be pointed and your palms facing. Be sure not to curve your spine but keep your back in a neutral position. Slowly raise your legs as shown in the top image. Your lower legs should be parallel with the ground.

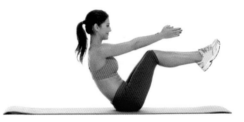

Exhale and twist your upper body to the right. Your arms should move towards the floor because of your body rotation.

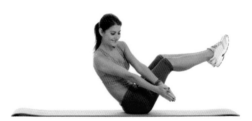

Return to the start position, and inhale. Repeat to the left to complete a full rep.

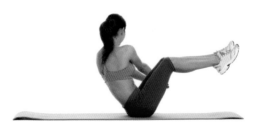

Bicycle kicks

This has been rated one of the top exercises for abs. Focus on proper form to start with, and take it slowly. Aim for quality until you are sure you are doing it right, then increase the speed.

Lie on your back on a mat. Extend your legs and raise your feet off the floor slightly. Keeping a neutral spine position, rest your hands behind your ears. Look straight up towards the ceiling.

Now bend your right leg to lift the knee towards the chest. At the same time, raise and twist your upper body slightly. You are aiming to touch your right knee with the elbow of the left arm.

Then extend the right leg and switch to bring up your left knee. Your upper body should twist in the other direction so that your left knee is aiming for the elbow of your right arm. Keep the move fluid but controlled. Your legs should mimic the movements of pedalling a bike. Your feet should not touch the floor until you have finished all your reps.

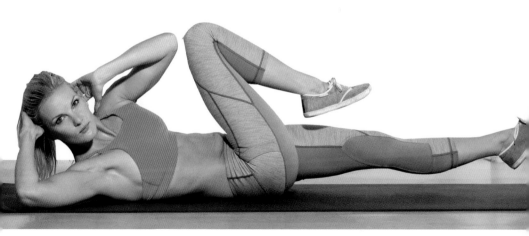

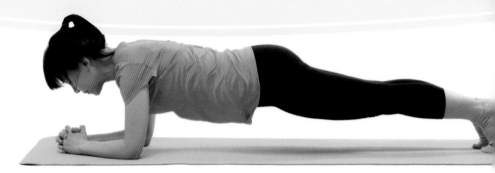

The plank

Love it or hate it, planking is an amazing discipline that strengthens your core and back, and can be modified to engage your arms, shoulders, glutes and hamstrings along the way.

Begin with a standard plank. Position yourself with your elbows bent and underneath your shoulders, legs outstretched and resting on your toes. Your feet should be hip-width apart. Squeeze your glutes and your core muscles to keep your body straight and flat. Ensure your bottom is tucked in, not sticking up in the air.

Many people plank with their arms outstretched instead of bent. Try both positions for 30 seconds. If you're new to this, you're guaranteed a wobble before the time is up! If you feel ready for a challenge, walk the plank – start in one position and swap to the other, elbows to hands, over and over again at a steady pace. Concentrate on keeping your hips and body as still as possible.

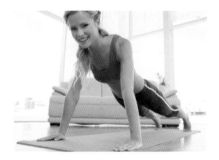

Look ahead!

Keep your head straight, gazing at a point on the floor about 30 centimetres beyond your hands. This will keep your neck and spine properly aligned.

Supersized plank

Once you can comfortably hold a plank for more than a minute, you can add in some variation. Raise one leg or one arm in the air and hold it without wobbling or rotating your pelvis. Holding your body straight will increase the intensity of the move.

Try planking with your legs on an exercise ball. Again, hold it tight and still without moving around.

Side plank

Up your game in a different way with a side plank. From a straight arm plank, press into your right hand, keeping it on the floor, and turn your body to face the wall. Rest your left foot on top or in front of your right foot and extend your left arm high into the air, stacking your hips so that they're level. Brace and hold for as long as you can, then swap to the other side.

You can add movements to your basic planks; turn to page 85 for a plank-based routine.

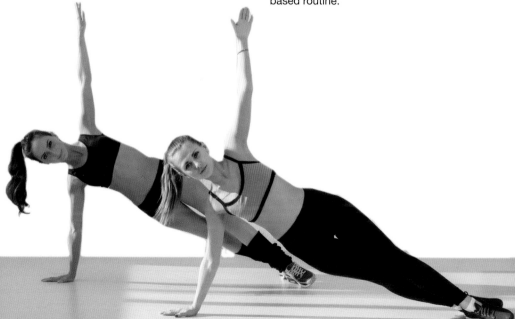

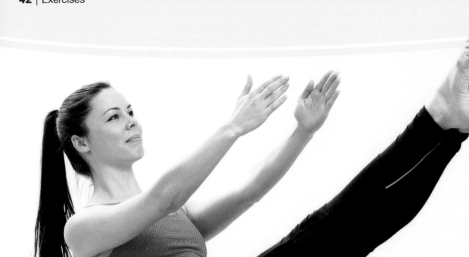

V-sit

Like so many of these exercises, this one can be done at home without any specialist equipment. Try it in front of the TV!

Sit on the floor with your legs outstretched. Pull in your core muscles, keeping a neutral spine position, and raise your legs off the ground to make a V shape. Extend your arms, palms facing.

Hold this position for several seconds, concentrating on keeping your abdominal muscles contracted. Keep breathing!

Slowly lower your legs, but just before they touch the floor, stop. Hold this position for a few more seconds. Repeat the whole movement for the desired number of reps.

Bird flaps

This is a variation on the V-sit. It relies on core stability to keep your body still while your arms move. It may seem easy, but don't be fooled.

Lie on the floor with your legs and arms outstretched. Engage your abs to push your lower back into the floor. Raise your feet so your legs are at a 45-degree angle.

Now lift up your upper back, using your stomach muscles to hold yourself so that your shoulder blades barely make contact with the floor. Keep this position and pump your arms up and down. The movement can be small but speedy, and keep your body stationary. If you begin to lose posture, bend your knees but keep your feet off the ground.

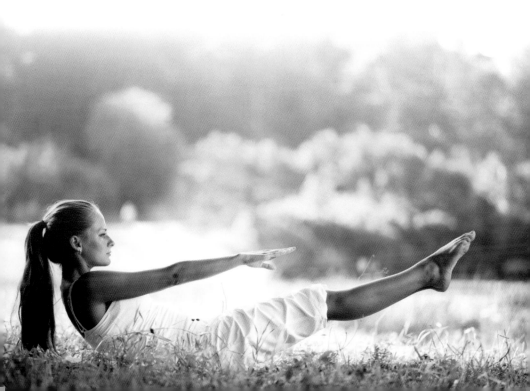

Circles and twists

These two simple exercises will work your abs and obliques, and help with hip flexibility.

Air circles

Lie on your back on a soft surface. Place your feet together, legs outstretched, arms by your side on the floor.

Engage your abs and lift your legs from the hip until they point to the ceiling. Aim for a 45-degree angle. Draw a large circle with your feet, toes pointed upwards, then repeat in the opposite direction. Also try this with your arms straight up in the air.

Heel twists

Kneel on an exercise mat and push your body off the ground so that your hips are raised above your knees. Rest your hands behind your head, elbows pointing out.

Keeping your hips still, twist your upper body to the left and reach your left hand to your left ankle. Bring the movement back to the centre, then repeat in the other direction.

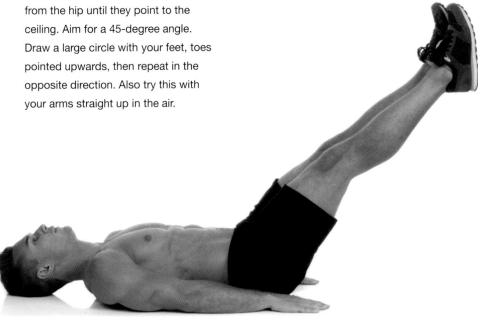

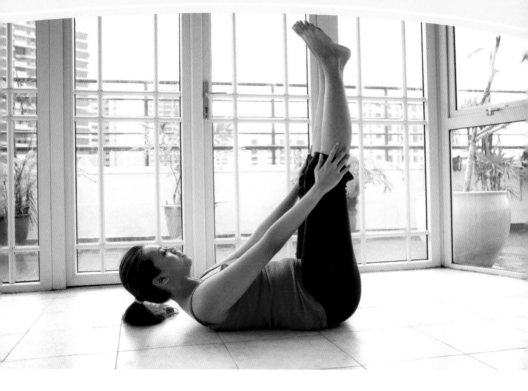

Double crunch

As you progress and get fitter, you can move on to more advanced movements. Unlike many muscle groups, you can work your abs every day – after all, they're the main ones holding you up all the time. Vary your standard crunches by adding in some alternatives.

Lie on your back and raise your legs so they are pointing straight up. Keep your feet flexed not pointed.

Lift your arms to point towards the ceiling. Now engage your abs to lift your upper body AND your hips off the floor, aiming to touch your toes.

Using your core muscles for control, slowly lower yourself back to the floor.

Remember, during this exercise, try to keep your spine in a neutral position.

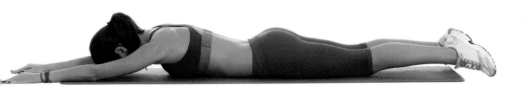

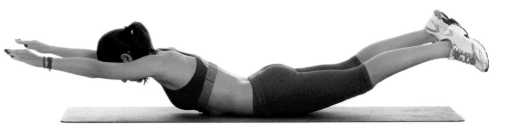

Superman!

This move might give you the abs of a superhero, but is named because of the pose you assume – like Superman flying through the air. It is good for back strength and engages your abs nicely.

Lie on your front on a mat or carpet. Stretch your arms out in front of you.

Inhale and lift your arms and legs off the ground, keeping them straight. You should feel floor contact only between your lower ribs, tummy and pelvis.

Hold for five seconds, then exhale as you lower yourself to the start position. If this is too hard for you, start with arms only, or try one arm and one leg on opposite sides.

Head position

As in previous exercises, keep your head stable by gazing at a point on the floor about 30 centimetres beyond your hands.

Climb-ups

You will need a resistance band or a strong scarf for this exercise.

Lie on the floor on your back. Loop the band around your feet. Raise both legs into the air. Straighten them as much as you can.

Hold the band in both hands and keep your feet flexed.

Now 'climb' up the band, hand over hand, using your stomach muscles to lift your upper body off the floor. Lower yourself back down gradually, repeating the hand over hand movement.
Do 10 reps.

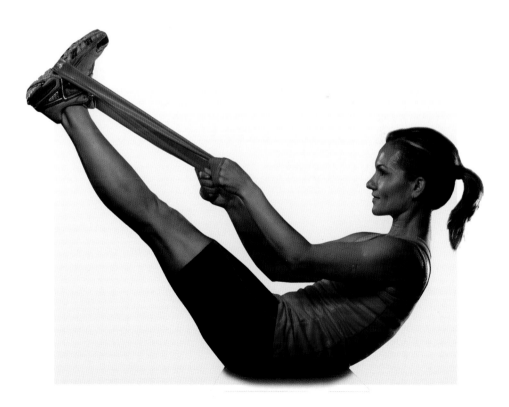

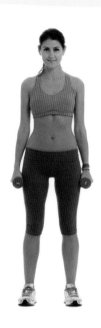

Side bends

It's time to get off the floor and do a standing abs exercise. This one works your obliques to shape your waist.

Stand with your feet shoulder-width apart and knees slightly bent. Hold a dumb-bell (or a can of food) in each hand, resting by your thighs.

Exhale and slide a weight down one leg as far as you can comfortably go. Imagine you are pivoting around your tummy button.

Inhale and return to the start position, keeping your hips stationary. Repeat on this side and then swap to the other side.

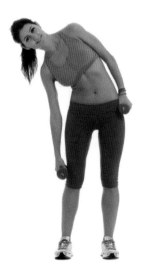

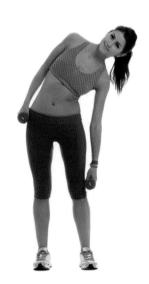

Deadbug

When you assume the position for this exercise you will see how it got its name! It really targets your six-pack muscles.

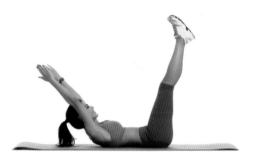

Lie on your back with your arms and legs stretched up to the ceiling. Flatten your back to the floor and squeeze your bottom muscles tight.

Now lower your left arm and right leg, making sure the movement is smooth but controlled. Don't touch the floor at the lowest point. Be sure to keep your back pressed flat or in a neutral position.

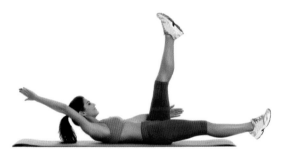

Return to the start position and then repeat with the right arm and left leg to complete one rep. If you find that your lower back lifts, try perfecting the exercise with knees bent, stretching them out straight instead of raising and lowering them.

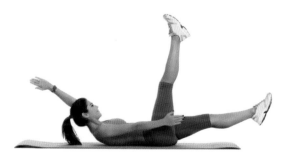

Floor Work: Upper Body

As you get into shape for summer, don't forget your flip side. There are certain 'back bits' you can't easily see in the mirror that may need toning and slimming to allow you to don strapless tops and skinny vests with confidence. And of course you'll want lean, firm arms for all the short sleeves you'll be wearing. Many arm exercises also work the shoulders, which will firm the bits of body around your upper back.

There are a variety of exercises here that can be done at home or in the gym with minimal equipment. However, there are so many variations in the ways you can hold and lift that only a selection are shown here.

You may also feel that your upper body would benefit from gym sessions using the weights machines. Always consult a gym professional before beginning to use the equipment. He or she will instruct you on how to use each one and what to do for your own particular goals.

Working together

Many people choose to add an arm movement to a movement that works another part of the body, such as a squat or a lunge, instead of spending precious time standing still and working only the arms.

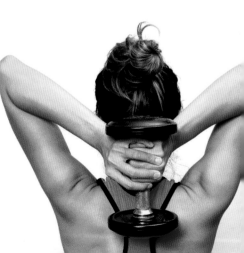

Bicep curls

These are a must for well-defined arms, but don't worry about looking like a body builder. It takes long hours, a strict-diet regime and total dedication to get bulging biceps, so a few reps in your workout aren't going to make your muscles pop!

The move is a simple one, which is why it can be combined with lower body exercises. Stand with your back straight, chest held high and stomach engaged.

Hold a pair of dumb-bells or other suitable weights (try cans of food) in your hands. Extend your arms by your sides and turn them so the palms of your hands face forwards.

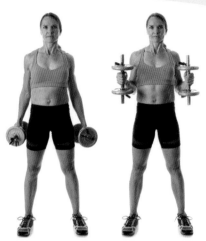

Keep your upper arms still, elbows tucked in to your sides, and bend your elbows to raise the weights to your shoulders. Slowly lower the weights back to your sides.

This move can also be done with your palms facing backwards (facing your body) or inward (thumbs forwards). The latter are known as hammer curls and place less stress on the wrists.

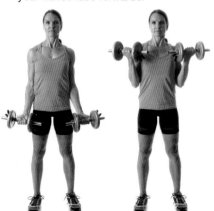

What weight?

Many women have relatively weak arms that need building up. Start with a 2 kg or 3 kg weight but quickly move up to 5 kg if you don't feel the strain by the end of your reps.

Tricep dips

If you want to avoid saggy underarms, you will need to work your triceps. Dips work your arms, your back and shoulders, using your own bodyweight. Find a stable surface to perform this exercise, such as a sturdy chair or coffee table.

Sit on the edge of the bench (or chair or table) and grip the edge with your hands at your sides. Curl your fingers over the edge if possible. Stretch your feet out in front of you.

Slide yourself forwards so that you are supporting your own weight. Your heels should be resting on the ground and your elbows should be pointing backwards. Bend the elbows slightly.

Now bend your elbows further to slowly lower your body towards the ground. Keep your back straight and ensure your elbows bend backwards, not out to the sides. Your bottom should nearly, but not quite, touch the floor.

Push back up until your elbows are nearly straight but not locked. Repeat.

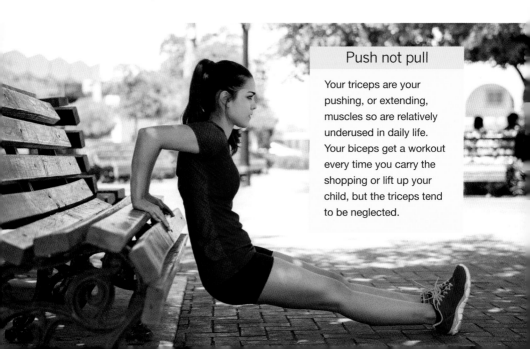

Push not pull

Your triceps are your pushing, or extending, muscles so are relatively underused in daily life. Your biceps get a workout every time you carry the shopping or lift up your child, but the triceps tend to be neglected.

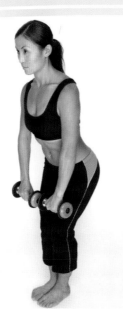 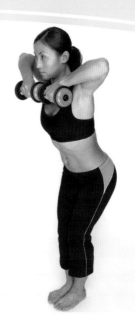

Upright rows

Target your shoulders with this exercise. It can be done on its own, weight-free, as you work on other movements such as step-ups, but is more beneficial if done using weights.

To perform the move on its own, stand with your feet at shoulder-width and knees loose, not locked. Keep your back straight and your chest high.

Hold your weights – a barbell or kettlebell in both hands, or a dumb-bell in each hand – palms downwards.

Bend your arms to lift your hands towards your chin, in a rowing motion. At the top of the movement, your elbows should be higher than your shoulders and pointing out to the sides. Lower and repeat.

Rows can be done one handed to work your lower back as well as your arms and shoulders. Rest one arm and one knee on a bench and hold the weight in your free hand. Keep your back naturally arched and bend your elbow to raise it to the ceiling, lifting the weight. Your upper arm should be parallel to the floor. Slowly lower and repeat.

Raises – lateral and front

These simple moves will work your shoulders. Use weights or dumb-bells if you have them, or improvise with anything weighted that has a handle. Paint tins or kids' buckets with stones in will do the trick!

Stand with your feet shoulder-width apart, knees soft, back straight, arms by your sides. Hold the weights with your palms facing inwards. Inhale.

Keep your body still and lift your arms up to shoulder height. Allow your elbows to bend slightly and your hands to tilt forwards a little. Exhale as you lift. Hold the lift for a moment, then lower your arms and repeat.

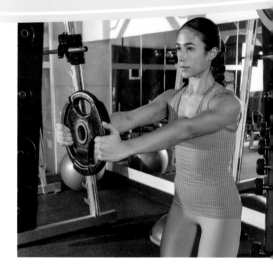

Front raises

Assume the same start position but with your hands in front of your thighs, palms towards you. Repeat the exercise but this time, raise the weights in front of your body. You can also perform this with a single weight such as a heavy book held with both hands.

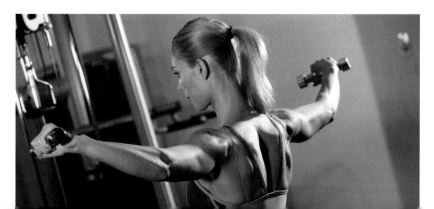

Tricep kickbacks

Yet again, you will need to push against a weight to fully work your tricep muscles. Concentrate on performing these properly before you increase reps or weight.

Hold a weight in one hand and lean forwards. You can rest the other hand on your thigh for support. Look slightly forwards, not behind. Bend your elbow and lift the weight to the starting position. Your upper arm should be in line with your back, elbow tucked in. Inhale.

Now exhale and use your triceps to straighten the elbow to extend your arm behind you. Hold, then return to the start position.

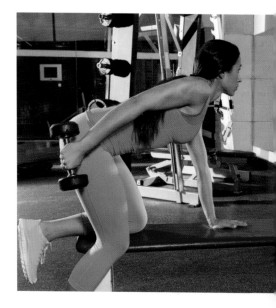

Overhead triceps extension

Stand with a weight held in both hands above your head. Keep your feet shoulder-width apart and knees soft. Squeeze your arms to your ears and bend your elbows to lower the weight behind your head. Engage your triceps to lift the weight back to the start position.

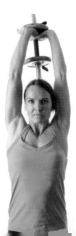 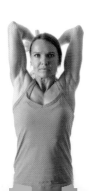

Press-ups

Don't be afraid of press-ups! They really will help to get your arms and shoulders in shape, faster than almost any other exercise. They will work your chest and abs, too. The key to success is a strong core to keep your body in position during the move.

Lie face down on the floor and place your hands next to your shoulders. Push your body off the ground with your fingers facing forwards. Raise yourself onto your toes, legs straight, and hold yourself securely above the ground. Pull your bottom down so that your back is straight.

Now inhale and lower your chest towards the ground by bending your elbows. Keep your abs and bottom braced so that you aren't trying to lower a wobbly mass instead of a good, solid body! Raise your head slightly so that your chin, not your nose, is heading to the ground.

Go as low as you can, then push back up using upper arm strength. Remember to stay strong, and keep your bottom and back flat. Congratulations! You just did a press-up!

Foot position

Your feet can be together or apart for press-ups. Choose what suits you best. The wider they are, to just beyond shoulder-width distance apart, the more stable you will be.

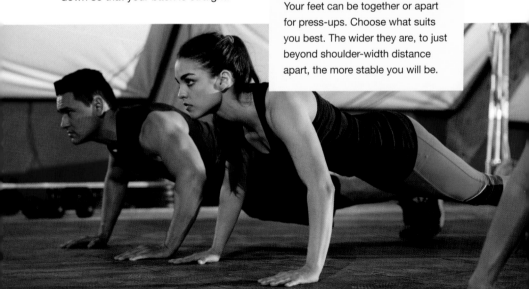

Too hard?

Learn the technique by doing press-ups against a wall standing up, or against a raised surface like the edge of a table. Progress to floor press-ups on your knees instead of with straight legs.

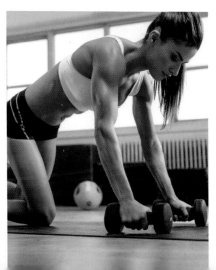

Super press-ups

Once you've mastered the basics, mix it up a little to avoid boredom, work different muscles, to push the boundaries of what you can do. Increase or decrease the distance between your hands to see the effects. Press-ups can be done on one arm or one leg, with your feet raised on a bench, or with your hands resting on weights or even a ball to increase instability and test your balance. Be careful with all of these if you have weak wrists.

Balls for biceps

The good old-fashioned medicine ball comes and goes, but it can be a great tool for your workout. If you're working at home, use the heaviest ball or similar object you can find, such as a doorstop.

Aim to do three minutes, repeating these three exercises without putting the ball on the floor at any point. Build up your time gradually. Stand with your feet a little way apart, knees soft, back straight.

Start by performing bicep curls (see page 51), holding the ball between both hands. Do ten curls, then hold the ball straight out in front of you. Keep your arms extended for a count of 30, then move straight into shoulder presses. Hold the ball at your chest, and press it up to the ceiling. Using all your arm strength, raise it above your head, then lower and repeat for a count of 20.

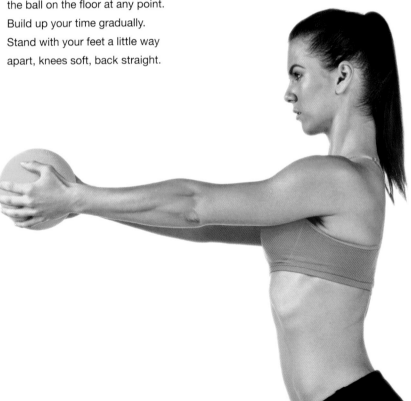

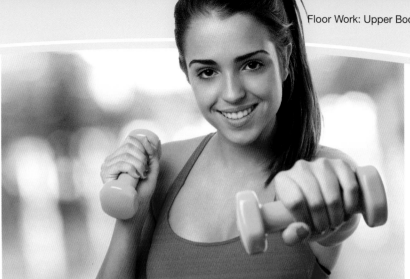

Ball slam

Imagine you're feeling a little tense. Let's harness that and use it to pound out some moves. The ball slam is especially good for your lateral muscles at the sides of your upper back.

Hold a medicine ball between both hands, feet shoulder-width apart. Inhale as you raise the ball above your head and rise up on your toes, extending to your full height.

Now use all your tension, rage, anger and power to bring down your arms and slam the ball hard into the ground near your feet. Squat down, back straight and legs bent, to pick up the ball and start again.

Punches

Punch away your stress and give your whole upper body a workout. Stand with one foot forwards, knees slightly bent. Hold your hands in front of your face with your elbows bent at right angles. Punch out with one arm. Straighten at the elbow and rotate so that your palm goes from facing inwards to facing down. Bring back that arm and repeat with the other arm. Aim to keep punching for at least 30 reps.

You can do this exercise with or without weights. Begin with cans of food or 2 kg dumb-bells.

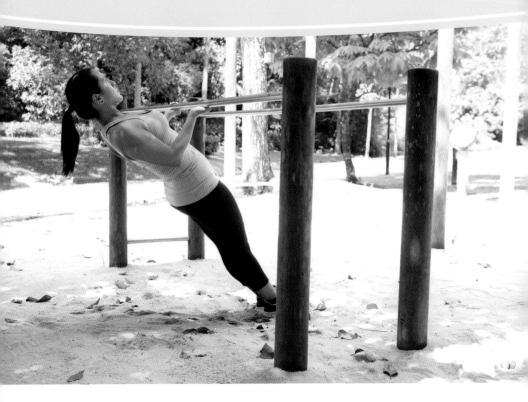

Pull-ups

Here's another exercise that may pose a challenge, especially if you're a woman with relatively low upper-body strength. Just start slowly and don't worry if you can only manage one or two pull-ups at first.

Start with Australian pull-ups, which are a bit like an inverted push-up. You will need a bar that is shoulder height or lower.

Position yourself underneath it with your legs straight, heels on the ground and hands holding onto the bar. Straighten your arms so you are lying back, supported beneath the bar. Experiment to see if you prefer an overhand or underhand grip.

Now, keeping your feet on the ground, bend your elbows to pull your chest to the bar. Keep your body straight so that it acts as the weight you're lifting with your arms. Lower back down and repeat.

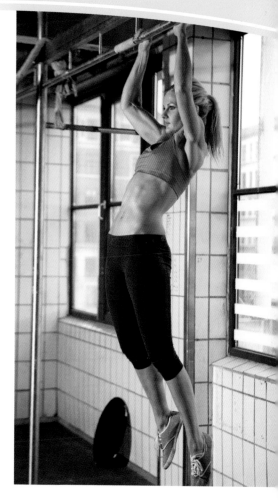

When you are capable of doing those, find a full height pull-up bar and hang from it. Learn to keep your body straight and taut without swinging. Slowly raise your legs to 90 degrees, so they are held straight out in front of you. Hold this position for as long as you can, but keep breathing!

The next stage is a chin-up. Grip the bar from the far side, with your fingers curled towards you, shoulder-width apart. Keep your body tight and use your arms to pull your head up to the bar, or above it if you can. Inhale as you lower yourself back down.

Now you can move on to a full pull-up. Grasp the bar the other way, fingers pointing away from you. Repeat the movement towards the bar. You may find it better to widen the gap between your hands a little.

Words of warning

Like press-ups, the key to success is to keep your core tight. Otherwise, you'll end up flapping and flailing like a fish. However, be aware that pull-ups are harder if you're carrying too much extra weight. Go easy on yourself and just try again as your summer fit plan kicks in and you get lighter and stronger.

Floor Work: Lower Body

As the days become longer, get ready for fabulous summer clothes by targeting your legs and bottom. These lower body workouts can be done either at home or in the great outdoors. Bodyweight exercises can be done anywhere, without specialist equipment, and the sheer joy of moving around in the sunshine will give you an added glow and boost your energy levels.

The important thing to remember with lower body exercises is to move slowly into position, then power out of the move, focusing on the muscles involved for the maximum burn. Squeeze your glutes and engage your core, while maintaining good posture to prevent back and joint injuries.

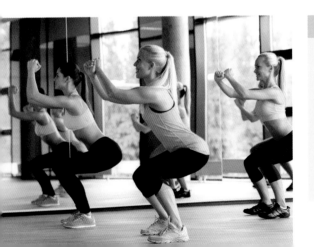

Fat-burning boost

The great news about targeting your lower body is that it contains some of the biggest muscles: the glutes and quads. Using these large muscle groups is an instant fat burner, upping your metabolic rate and burning more calories.

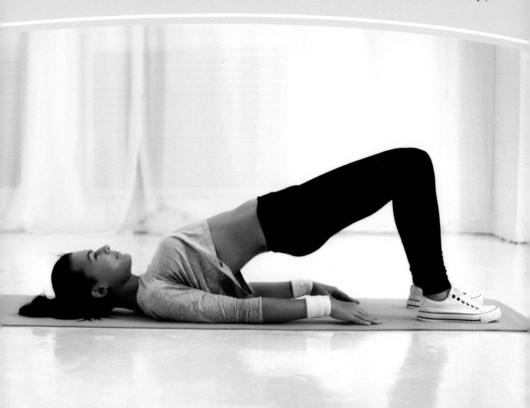

The bridge

This simple exercise works wonders on the backs of your legs and your bottom, and strengthens your back. You can do it anywhere, including in the ad breaks as you watch TV!

Lie on your back on a soft surface. Bend your knees and place your feet flat on the floor hip-width apart.

Raise your hips to lift them in line with your shoulders and knees. Hold this position for a count of five, then release down. Try to keep your torso still during the raised part of the exercise.

Modify the exercise by raising one leg in the bridge position. Lift your body as before, then pull one knee closer to your chest. Keep your hips square; don't rotate as you lift the knee.

Lunges

If you want to tone your thighs, this is a great exercise. Once again, it can be done anywhere, any time, and no specialist equipment is needed. Perfect your technique so you don't strain your joints.

Step forwards on your right leg so that your left leg is extended behind you. Bend your knee so that your right knee forms a 90-degree angle, ensuring that it remains above your ankle. Don't push too far forwards or twist to the side.

Keep your upper body straight, shoulders back, and look ahead, not down. Engage your core and drop your back knee towards the floor, rolling onto the toes of your back foot. Hold for a second, then press into your heels to push back to the start position.

Ease the strain

If you find that lunging strains your knees, take smaller steps.

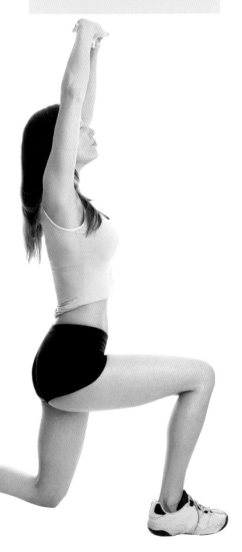

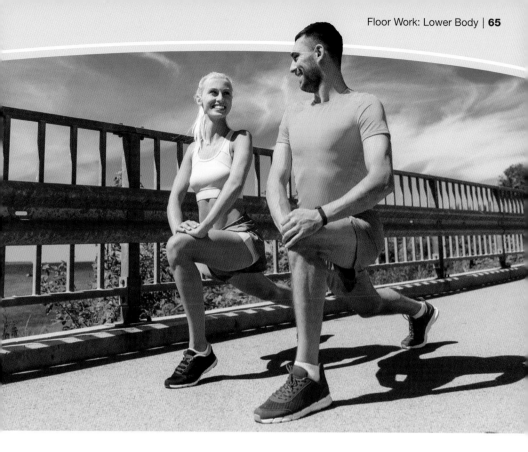

There are several variations you can try to keep boredom at bay and target extra muscles. If balance is a problem, walk as you lunge, and work your hip flexors that little bit extra. Or try reverse lunges; step back instead of forwards to engage your brain in a way that is different from everyday motion.

Side lunges reduce the risk of knee injury and work your lower body muscles in a different way.

Begin with your feet together, then take a large step sideways. Lunge towards the floor as you move. As before, make sure your bent knee does not go past your foot. Keep your other leg straight.

Push through the foot of your bent leg to press back to the start position. Take it up a notch by placing your front foot on a step, or by holding dumb-bells and adding a bicep curl.

Squats

Many of the best moves use your body weight to present resistance. Squats are one of the staple exercises to get the bottom and thighs you're after. Just be sure that you use the proper technique to avoid straining.

For a basic squat, stand with your feet shoulder-width apart. Raise your arms straight in front of you, palms down, and look ahead.

Bend your knees and lower your bottom towards the floor, keeping your back straight. Push your hips back to ensure your knees stay above your feet.

Now press into your heels and use your legs to thrust back to a standing position. Repeat slowly, aiming to go as low as you can, rather than as fast as you can.

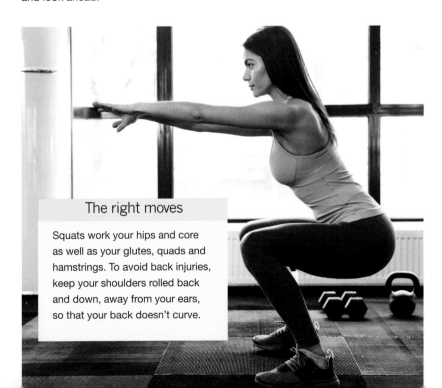

The right moves

Squats work your hips and core as well as your glutes, quads and hamstrings. To avoid back injuries, keep your shoulders rolled back and down, away from your ears, so that your back doesn't curve.

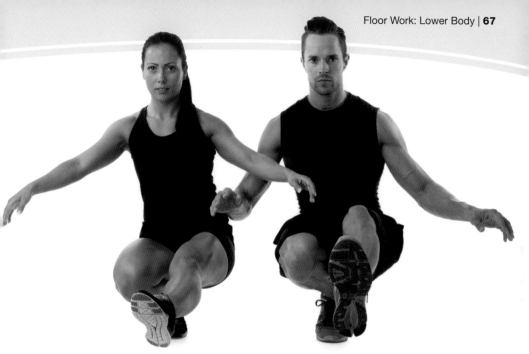

Pistol squat

A one-legged squat will put your strength and balance to the test, but don't try it until you can perform lots of normal squats with good posture.

Start as before but lift your left foot off the floor slightly before you begin the downwards movement. As you lower your bottom, lift your left leg straight out in front of you.

Wall sit

Here's another tricky one that uses the quads to hold a squat position. Stand with your back against a smooth wall, feet shoulder-width apart and roughly 60 centimetres away from the wall.

Slide your back down the wall until your thighs are parallel to the ground, knees above your ankles. Adjust your feet if you need to. Keep your back flat against the wall and hold the position until your thighs begin to burn. You may only last 10 seconds to begin with, but you should work your way to staying there for more than a minute. Don't rest your hands on your thighs!

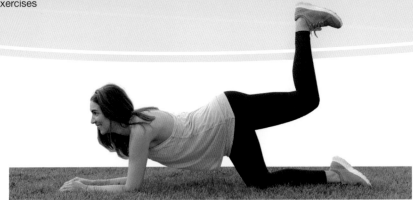

Kneeling leg raise

This exercise targets your upper legs and your bottom.

Start by kneeling on your knees and elbows. Position your elbows directly below your shoulders, and your knees below your hips. Pull in your stomach and keep your back strong.

Raise your left heel towards the ceiling, keeping your knee bent so that your leg forms an L-shape. Contract your glutes to lift the foot a tiny bit higher, and pulse for a count of five. Lower your knee back to the floor and repeat on the other leg.

Donkey kick

Kneel on your hands and knees. Work your bottom and legs some more by keeping one leg bent and on the floor while raising the other and pushing the foot out to straighten the leg as you lift. Keep your core braced. Lower and repeat, and then switch legs.

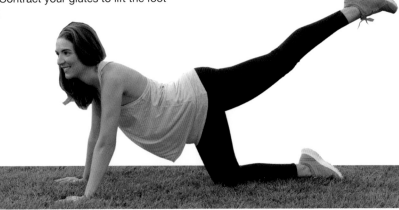

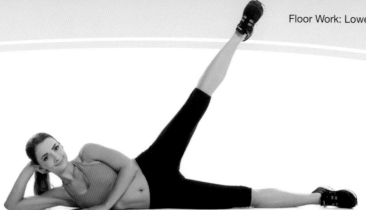

Side leg raise

Strengthen and shape your outer thigh with this move. You can add extra resistance by linking your feet with a resistance band. Change the move slightly to work the inner thigh with a lower leg raise.

Lie on your side on the floor and prop up your head on your elbow. Rest your other hand in front of you to keep you stable. Extend your legs but keep your feet flexed.

Engage your core and slowly lift your top leg towards the ceiling. Don't allow your hips to rotate. At the top of the move, pulse your leg upwards a tiny bit more for 10 lifts. Lower your leg and repeat before switching sides.

To switch to the inner thigh, cross your top leg over with bent knee so your foot is on the floor in front of your other knee. Now lift the bottom leg off the floor, keeping your torso still; the range of movement is obviously much smaller because of your position. Lower the leg and repeat, or pulse at the top of the move as before.

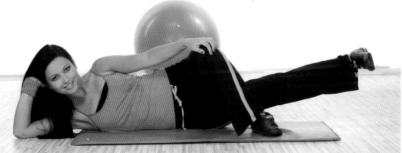

Step-up with knee raise

The action of climbing upwards works your lower body. Simply taking the stairs or walking uphill will tone your bottom more than exercising on level ground. Try the following move to improve your balance and co-ordination at the same time.

Stand facing a step, bench or any other item that will take your weight when you step onto it. Your feet should be almost together.

Step up to put your right foot on top of the bench. Raise your body using the strength in this right leg. As you reach the top of the movement, lift your left knee to bring it as high as you can.

Swing the left leg back down to stand back on the floor. Step down with your right, tap the foot on the ground and repeat the action. Swing your arms and build up a marching rhythm through the reps.

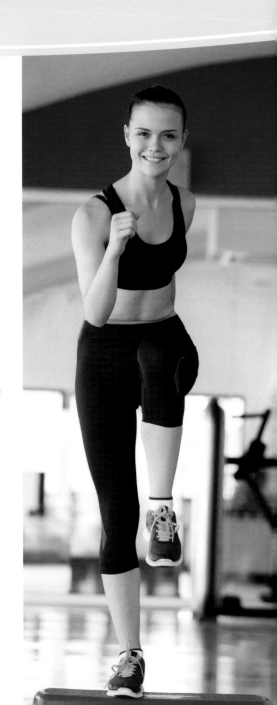

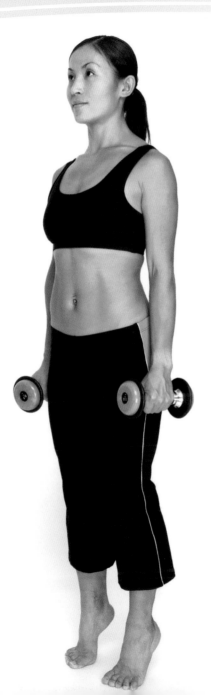

Calf raises

Sometimes the smallest movements are all that is needed to target specific muscles. The following exercise focuses on your calf muscles for shapely lower legs.

Stand with your feet together, flat on the floor. Slowly rise up onto your toes, lifting your heels off the ground. Keep your knees straight. Hold for a second and then lower your heels back down.

To increase the range of movement here, perform the exercise standing on a step, allowing your heels to drop below the edge of the step holding on to a banister for safety. Or hold onto the back of a chair and squat down, then raise and lower your heels.

If you feel this is becoming too easy, move onto single-legged raises and build on your balance and strength.

Single leg deadlift

Hamstrings can be a problem area for many people, especially keen sportsmen and women. Get them into shape for rounders, and shorts!

Practise this move first without weights, and then try it holding a kettlebell or bar weights. Stand on one leg and bend that knee slightly.

Rotate at the hip, bending forwards until your body is parallel to the floor. Raise your free leg behind you, toes pointed downwards. Keep your chest firm and your back straight. Let your arms hang towards the ground. Now return to the starting position. Repeat for the required number of reps, then swap legs.

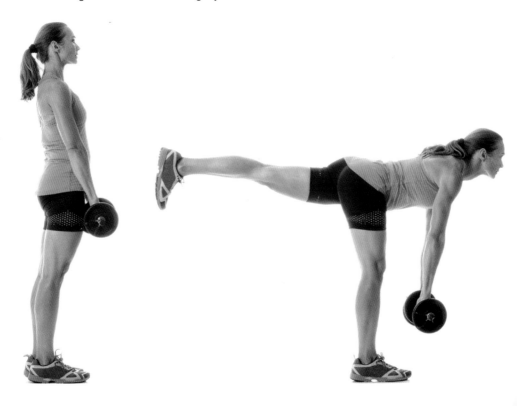

Inchworm

Done properly, this exercise has all the grace and elegance of the yoga movements it is channelling. However, don't worry if yours looks slightly more cumbersome; it is named after a bug, after all! It will help to strengthen and lengthen your hamstrings.

Begin in a standing position with your feet close together. Bend over with your legs straight and put your hands flat on the floor, as close to your feet as you can.

Walk your hands forwards, left and then right, keeping your hips bent but your legs straight. Keep moving forwards to increase the gap between your hands and feet.

Eventually your hands will be so far forwards that you are in a plank position. Now take alternate steps with your left and right feet, to bring them back towards your hands. Keep your legs straight the whole time.

Compound Moves

So far, your exercises have focused mainly on one part of the body, to sculpt and tone specific areas. These are sometimes known as isolation exercises. Strictly speaking, isolation exercises work just a single muscle group. However, that rarely happens: even a simple bicep curl involves other muscles in the arms and also works the back, shoulders and core.

It is possible to work on several muscle groups together, with compound moves that engage your whole body. Not only does that help to get more body parts in shape, it also means that different areas of your body develop at a similar rate, to keep your body proportions the same. These compound moves help you do more work in less time and mimic everyday activities and sports that involve multiple movements. Compound moves build muscle fast, increase your overall strength, ramp up your heart rate and burn extra calories.

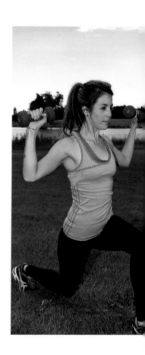

Don't be a lightweight

Add weights to your basic moves to increase their effect, and ensure you are lifting enough weight to make a difference. If you finish an exercise and could easily have done more reps, it's time to use slightly heavier weights.

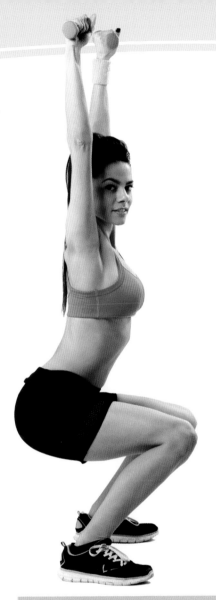

Press squats

Here is a simple variation on the squat that will work your arms as well as your legs. Use dumb-bells or, if you don't have any, cans of food or plastic 1-litre bottles filled with water.

Prepare to perform a squat as described on page 66. Hold a weight in each hand, above your shoulders – roughly level with your ears. Keep your elbows out to the sides.

Squat down with the weights by your ears, and then push out of the movement using your thighs. At the same time as your body rises, press the weights up into the air over your head.

Bring the weights back down to ear level as you lower yourself into the next squat. Take it slow and steady so that the move is done with precision.

Personal preference

Don't be afraid to rearrange a move so that it works for you. If your co-ordination means that you're happier doing the arm press on the downward move, do so.

Squat thrusts

This exercise is pretty old school, but it is effective. You should feel tired by the end of your reps, as the heart works harder to push blood to your muscles.

Begin with your hands on the floor, shoulder-width apart, arms and legs straight, as though you are about to do a press-up, as shown below.

Keeping your arms still, jump your feet in towards your hands, knees bent, so you are in a tuck position.

Now jump your feet backwards again to return to the start position. If you like, you can add in a press-up at this stage to work yourself even harder.

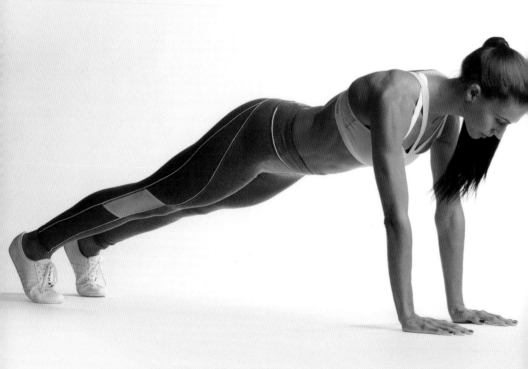

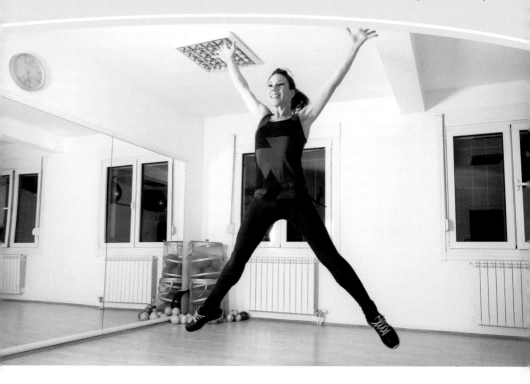

Burpees

Burpees require space, so make sure there is plenty of room to jump before you begin. Burpees use the squat thrust with a jump added in.

Start in a standing position. Squat down and place your hands on the ground in front of you, shoulder-width apart.

Kick your feet back, taking the weight on your hands, until your legs are fully extended. Keep your arms straight with your shoulders above your hands.

Jump your feet back to the start position in one movement, pulling in your knees. Raise your shoulders to the upright position and push with your feet to jump up in the air. Push through your legs until they are straight, and reach for the ceiling with your hands. If you prefer, do a star jump at this point: open your arms and legs wide to make a star shape.

Repeat in a flowing motion, bringing your arms down and going straight into the next squat.

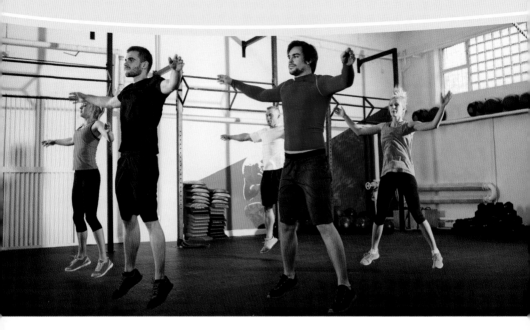

Jumping jacks

Many compound moves are high intensity, explosive moves (often referred to as plyometrics). Do them with a smile on your face!

Stand up straight with your feet together and arms by your sides. Now simply jump into a 'star' position, with your arms outstretched past your ears and legs in a wide stance, feet on the floor. Jump back to the start position and repeat, as fast as you can.

Add in an extra burn by squatting when you are in the star position and touching the floor between your feet with one hand. Keep the other arm pointing to the ceiling to make your torso twist.

Plyometrics for power

Most plyometrics are reminiscent of playground games: hopping, skipping and jumping. Your muscles are required to exert maximum force in short bursts. Plyometrics are great training for sports such as netball, basketball, tennis and volleyball.

Lunge shuffle

While your heart rate is up, try this basic move with a plyometrics twist to keep you in the cardio zone.

Lunge to the right (see page 65). Then reach down with your left arm to touch the ground between your feet.

Now push through your right heel to centre your bodyweight. With bent knees, shuffle two steps to the left, and then lunge again to the opposite side.

Keep repeating this movement for 30 seconds, constantly swapping legs and side-stepping in between lunges.

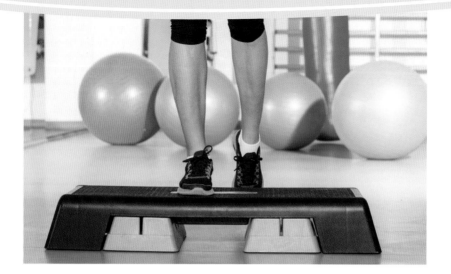

Forward jumps

If you're in the mood for a playful workout that really works up a sweat, include some jumping moves. Use a solid, secure raised surface. An aerobics step is ideal, as you can raise the height as you improve, but a single stair or a curb works well. Simply stand on the lower surface, feet slightly apart and knees bent. Power through your legs, ankles and feet to jump onto the higher surface, and then jump back down. Use your arms to provide extra thrust as you jump higher.

Forward hops

Change forward jumps into forward hops by carrying out the move on one leg. This will vastly improve your balance and work on your core stability.

Land lightly

Jumping movements are high impact so can take their toll on your joints. Be sure to land softly on the balls of your feet, absorbing the impact by bending your knees slightly. If you have weak knees or ankles, take it down a notch by stepping instead of jumping.

Scissor jumps

Begin in a forward lunge position (see page 64) with your left foot forwards, knee bent. After you lower your back leg, push up hard and fast with both legs to jump into the air. Swap legs in mid-air so that you land with your right leg forward.

Lateral jumps

Use a narrow hurdle such as an upturned book or a rolling pin rested on two tins. Stand to one side with your feet almost together. Bend at the knees and power up, jumping sideways to clear the hurdle. Land softly at the other side and then jump back immediately.

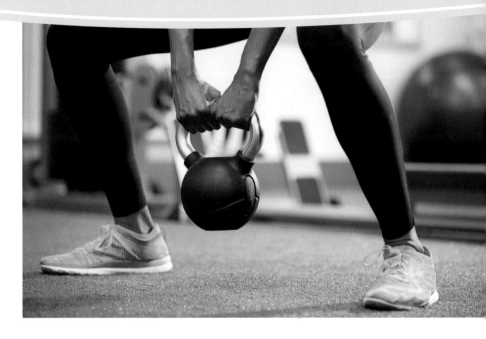

Kettlebell swing

Today's lifestyle sees many of us spending large parts of the day in a sitting position. Use a kettlebell swing to open up your frame from seated to extended, at the same time as working your legs, bottom and core.

Start by holding a weight with both hands. Your feet should be shoulder-width apart. Swing your arms to raise the weight to shoulder height, arms straight, and then lower it back to the resting position. When you raise your arms, make sure that you squeeze your glutes and thrust your hips forwards. Allow momentum, not your arms, to lift the weight.

Home-made weights

Instead of dumb-bells, you can use cans of food and as you progress to heavier weights, fill large (2.2 litre) milk cartons with water or sand. Make sure you screw the lid on tightly!

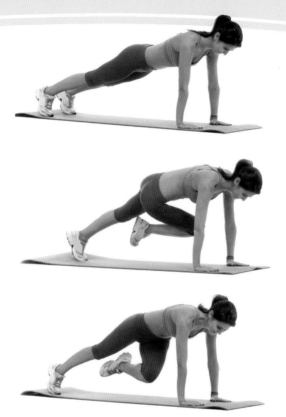

Mountain climber

Hit the floor for this high-powered workout move that uses just about every muscle that you might want to shape and tone.

Lie face down and raise yourself into a press-up position as you exhale. Your arms should be straight and your legs stretched out behind you, resting on your toes. Inhale and ensure your body forms a nice straight line.

Lift your right foot and bend your right knee until it nearly reaches your chest as you exhale. Inhale and push it back out straight and return your toes to the floor. Repeat with your left leg.

Repeat this movement over and over again. Start slowly but try to get faster once you are familiar with the actions involved. If you want to keep it low-impact, twist at the top of the movement to take the knee across your chest.

High knees

This exercise is like running on the spot, but with an exaggerated knee movement. It's great for warming up or keeping your heart-rate up between floor exercises.

Stand with your feet hip-width apart. Lift your left knee towards your chest, as high as you can. Lower it, and raise your right knee instead. Swing your arms to raise the opposite arm to leg.

Start slowly to combine a steady rhythm with a good high-knee action. Then raise onto your toes and speed up the leg movements until you are driving hard off the ground with each knee raise.

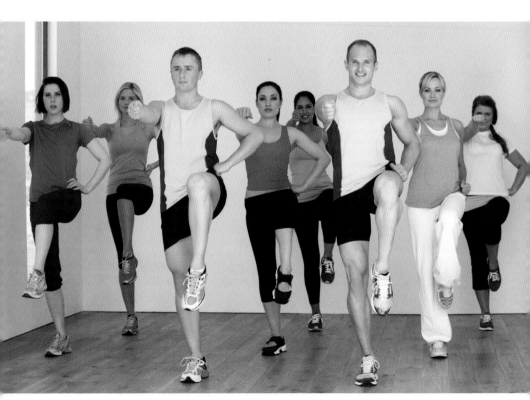

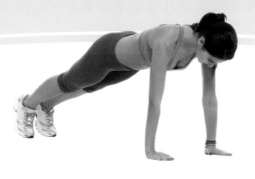

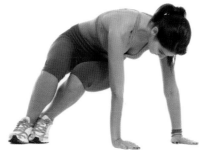

Jumping plank

Static planks are great
for your core and abs
but this version involves
jumps to work you harder
and raise your heart rate.
Assume a plank position with your
arms outstretched as shown in the
top image. Brace your toes against the
floor and jump into a forwards knee
bend, bringing your knees forwards.
As you move, twist at the waist to push
your knees out, past the level of your
elbow, as shown in the second image.
Both feet should be planted on the
floor behind your right hand.

Jump back to the starting position and
repeat on the left-hand side (bottom
image). As with previous moves, start
slowly to get used to the action, and
then speed up the whole sequence to
get your heart pumping.

Routines and Circuits

Chosen properly, the right combination of exercises will work on several levels: raising your heart rate for a cardio workout, and targeting various muscle groups for an all-over stretch and tone. You can achieve this with only a small number of carefully selected moves. Don't worry that you're not going all-out to work every muscle group with their own session; after all, if you went for a swim you wouldn't worry that you're limiting your workout.

These routines are best done in combination with a trip to the gym on subsequent days. And make sure you stretch and cool down once you're finished.

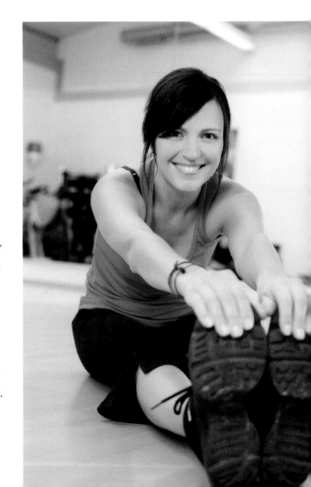

Super abs countdown combo

If you only have 15 minutes to spare for your daily dose of exercise, try this combo. It contains only two moves but burns fat fast, boosts your metabolism and works a whole range of muscles. You will need a kettlebell or dumb-bell, or a suitable home-made substitute.

Move 1 is the kettlebell swing, as described on page 82. Start with 10 reps, and then swap to move 2.

Move 2 is the squat thrust, as described on page 76. Again, do 10 reps, and then go straight back to move 1.

Don't rest in between moves, but lose one rep each time you swap – so that you count down 10, 9, 8 and so on until you do a single rep of each. In total, you will have done 110 reps, but hopefully without getting bored. Of course, you can begin with a higher number of reps as you improve.

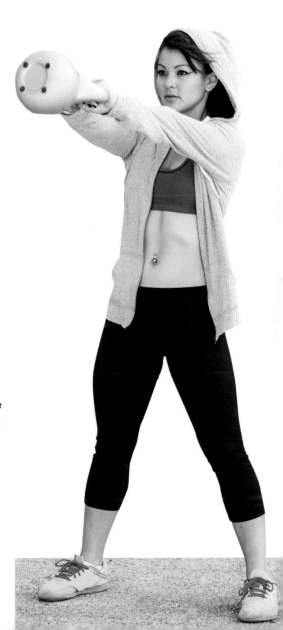

Plank routines

If you have become a planking pro, up your game even more with a selection of plank-based exercises. Begin with 6 reps (6 per side for the appropriate movements) and build up gradually as you become stronger and stronger.

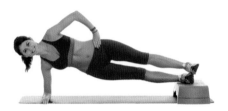

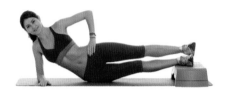

Side crunches – Begin in a side plank position on your right elbow, left arm extended upwards. Bend your left arm and crunch forwards and down with your left elbow, as if you are threading a needle through the space beneath your body. Straighten up and repeat. As you progress, do the movement on a fully extended arm, touching elbow to elbow as you crunch. Keep it slow and controlled.

Side raises – Again, start in a side plank position but this time raise your feet by placing them on a step. Ensure your feet are stacked on top of each other, and your elbow is directly under your shoulder. Now lower your body so that your hip grazes the ground. Raise it back to the starting position. This is very challenging and really engages your obliques.

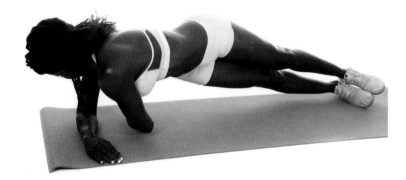

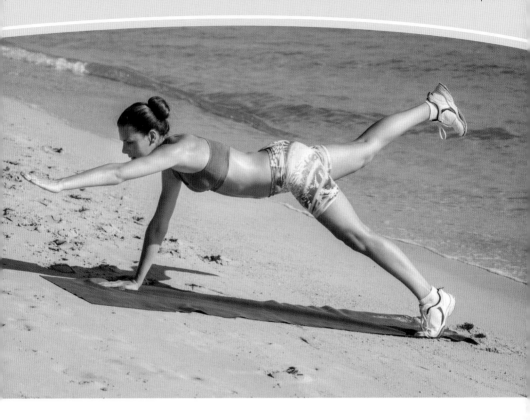

Plank raises – Start in a full plank position with extended arms. Look about 30 centimetres beyond your hands, keep your core super strong and raise your left arm. Now raise your right leg off the ground and try to keep stable. Lower your arm and leg to the start position and repeat with the other arm and leg. You will gain extra strength from this move by holding the balance.

Press-up planks – Begin in a press-up position near the ground. Push up to the extended arms stage of a press-up but as you rise, transfer your weight to your left hand. Turn into a side plank with your left arm straight and your right arm raised. Let your right foot sit on top of your left foot so both feet are stacked. Lower yourself back down and begin the press-up movement again, but this time turn to the opposite side for the side plank.

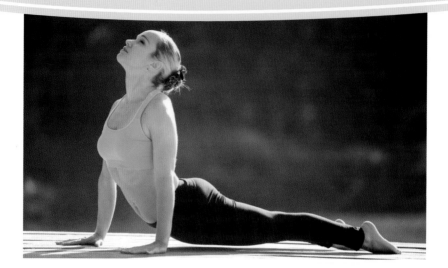

Stretch Routine

Use some classic yoga moves to stretch and tone, and give your core a boost. This routine is wonderful for a summer morning and can be done even when you are on holiday.

Kneel on a mat with your hands on the floor below your shoulders, arms straight. Inhale and curve your spine, pushing your tummy button down and your chin and tailbone up. Exhale and round your back upwards, chin to chest. Repeat for six breaths.

Inhale and step forwards with your left foot to place it between your hands. Keep your back leg outstretched,

bottom low. Exhale as you lift your left arm to the sky, twisting your body. Repeat on the other side and do three breaths each.

Step back into a plank position and inhale. Exhale as you lower yourself in a press-up. Repeat for six breaths.

Lower your body to the floor and inhale. Press your palms into the ground and exhale, pushing your upper body forwards and allow your thighs to lift. This is called the upward dog position, as shown. Hold for three breaths.

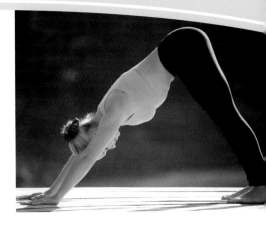

Exhale as you tuck your toes under to grip the floor and raise your bottom to the sky. Lower your head and straighten your arms to form an upside down V, as shown. Hold this downward dog for three breaths.

Step your feet to your hands and bend at the hips so your nose is touching your shins (or as close as you can comfortably get). Hold for two breaths. Inhale and move your feet to shoulder-width apart. Exhale and squat down so that your bottom drops towards the floor. Place your palms together in front of you, in a prayer position, and hold for three breaths.

Push up with your legs and inhale as you move your feet back together. Stay in a chair position, knees bent at

45 degrees, and exhale as you raise both arms to the sky. Hold for three breaths.

Inhale and stand tall, moving your weight onto your right foot. Exhale as you raise the left leg behind you, parallel with the floor (pictured). Feel the stretch through your body. Repeat on the other side and then bend at the hips again to touch your nose to your shins.

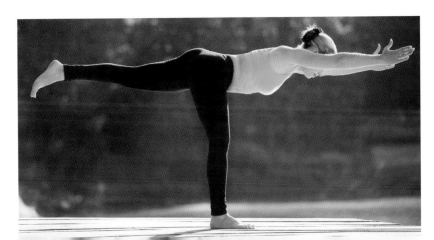

Get it Right

If you own a gym membership, the facility may offer a personal trainer to guide you with your technique, but what if you're going it alone? Start slow and steady to get into good habits before you go for the burn, whether it's on the road or in the pool. And be proud of what you're doing for your weight, fitness and stress levels.

Running

Running is a great way to burn calories and give your body a boost. Studies have found that it even adds years to life expectancy, improves your energy levels and lifts your spirits.

Tips for a great technique

Your whole body is involved in the action of running, so keep a check on where it's at. Look ahead, not down, and keep your chin tucked in. Your shoulders should be loose and low. Bend your elbows and swing your arms to match your stride. Don't clench your fists. Keep your body upright with your back straight, not hunched over. And listen to your feet; if they make a pounding sound then you're hitting the ground too hard. Land on the back of your foot and roll forwards to push off on your toes, with a spring in your step.

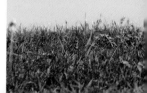

Myth busting

Don't believe what you hear
about running wrecking your
knees. Recent studies show that
it can strengthen the ligaments
and decrease the chances of
osteoarthritis. Losing weight will
also ease pressure on your joints.
However, it is very importantly
to properly stretch and cool
down after running to help
avoid muscular damage.

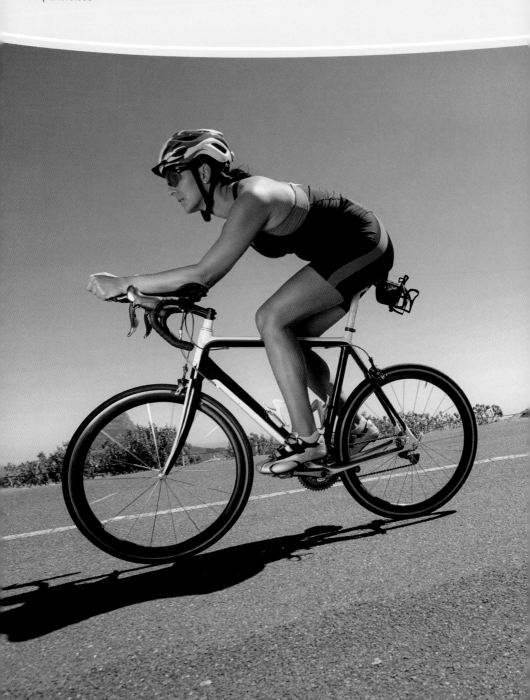

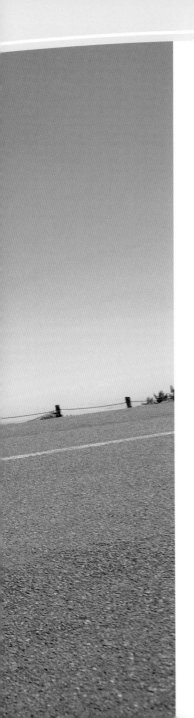

Cycle into summer

A bike ride is a brilliant way to enjoy the spring sunshine. A gentle cycle ride burns more calories than walking for the same length of time, and you can cover more miles to explore beyond the confines of your own neighbourhood. It is a low-impact form of exercise, and works your leg muscles in a way that will avoid injury and build muscle strength where it is most needed, to protect your joints.

Tips for a great technique
Concentrate on your foot position on the pedal. Keep your feet fairly flat with the toes pointing up ever so slightly. Push through the movement, from just before your foot hits the highest point in the rotation of the pedal. Make sure your saddle is at the optimum height. If your knees hurt at the back after a ride, your saddle may be too high. Pain at the front of the knee could be from your saddle being too low. And if your hands feel numb while you're riding, loosen your elbows. Relax your upper body for a better ride.

Mix it up

Although cycling is great for your heart and breathing, and strengthens your lower body, it doesn't do much for your core or upper body. Be prepared to lock up your bike and work on other areas at home or in the gym.

Swim happy!

Swimming is great low-impact exercise that raises your heart rate without you breaking into a sweat. It is ideal for getting started if your fitness levels are low, or you are carrying extra weight. Different strokes work different muscle groups, but your arms and legs will certainly benefit. Immersing yourself in the water has a soothing effect. As you gain in confidence and fitness, consider broadening your horizons with an open-water swim.

Tips for a great technique
A good stroke technique will speed up your swim to increase your work rate and burn more calories. You should glide through the water without too much splash. Swim one stroke until you begin to feel tired, and then switch to another stroke to work different muscles. Concentrate on your breathing; exhale under water so that you only have to inhale when your mouth is above water level. Don't let your feet sink too low in the water. Your body should be as flat in the pool as if you were planking on dry land.

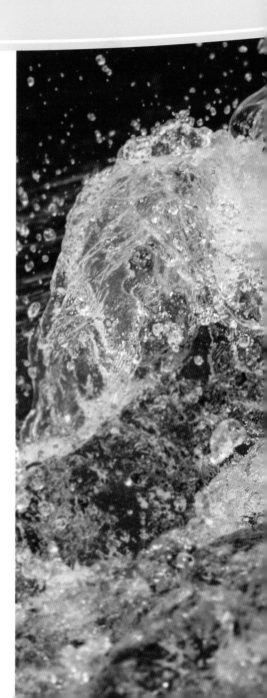

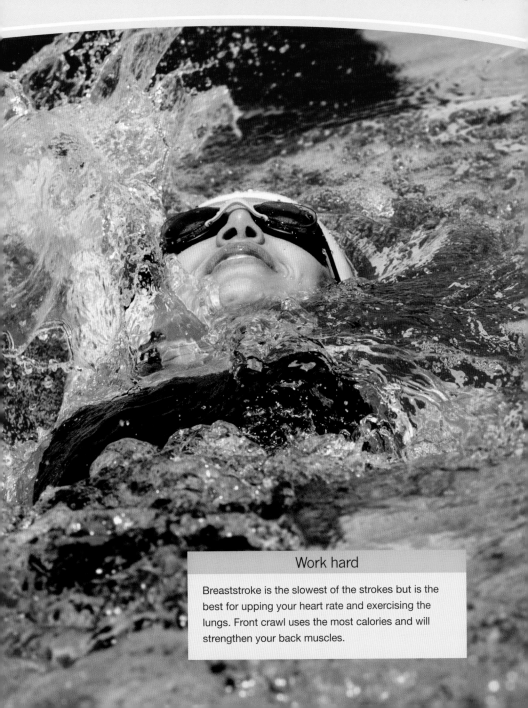

Work hard

Breaststroke is the slowest of the strokes but is the best for upping your heart rate and exercising the lungs. Front crawl uses the most calories and will strengthen your back muscles.

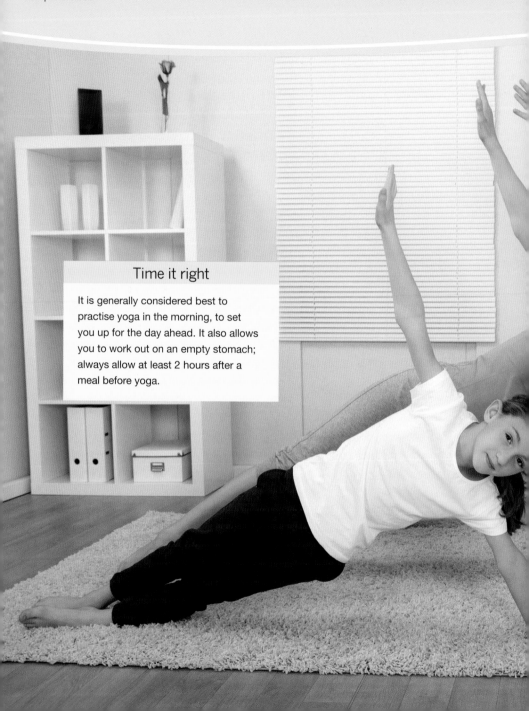

Time it right

It is generally considered best to practise yoga in the morning, to set you up for the day ahead. It also allows you to work out on an empty stomach; always allow at least 2 hours after a meal before yoga.

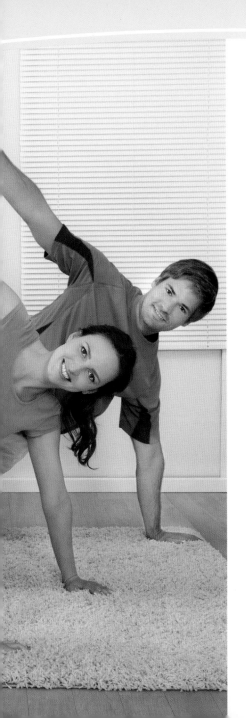

Yoga for you

Generally speaking, yoga will improve your flexibility and work your muscles, using your own bodyweight instead of reaching for the weights at the gym. There are several styles of yoga; investigate more than one to find one that suits your needs. Ashtanga is good for building strength and sculpting your muscles, while Bikram helps you work up a sweat, literally, as it is performed in a hot room. Yin yoga is more gentle but extremely good for gentle stretches to work your joints. Vinyasa classes use the basic poses to flow from move to move, so it feels more like a workout than some slower classes.

Tips for a great technique

The key to enjoying yoga is to know your own body. As a practice, it is an excellent way to become mindful of your own state, and to relieve the stresses of modern life. But don't fret if you're not as bendy as you'd like to be. Everyone's body is different, and you should work to your limits, not those of the person on the mat next to you. Take a few classes to learn the basics, and pay particular attention to your breathing, as guided by the instructor.

Pilates

Pilates is often bundled together with yoga, but there are differences. Pilates is a much younger discipline, and consists of a structured set of movements that link your mind and body in a healthy way. These movements will greatly increase your strength, and help to stretch and shape your muscles without bulking them up. Pilates is popular with dancers and is a great way to improve balance and posture, and really strengthen your core.

Tips for a great technique

It is important to relax into each movement, retaining strength without overdoing it. There should be a smooth flow from one movement to the next, with no jerkiness or tension. Pilates requires you to focus on your alignment and posture, in particular in the core area where a bundle of criss-crossing muscles protect your inner organs and spine. You will learn about 'centring' your core, drawing the muscles in your lower abs upwards and inwards towards your spine as you perform each movement. Listen to your body, though, and don't continue any action if it is causing pain rather than a stretch.

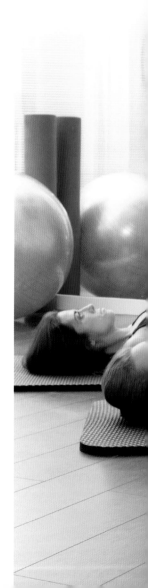

Breathe in and out

Breathing properly is a key concept in Pilates (and one that will help you in cardio workouts, too). Always breathe in through the nose and out through the mouth.

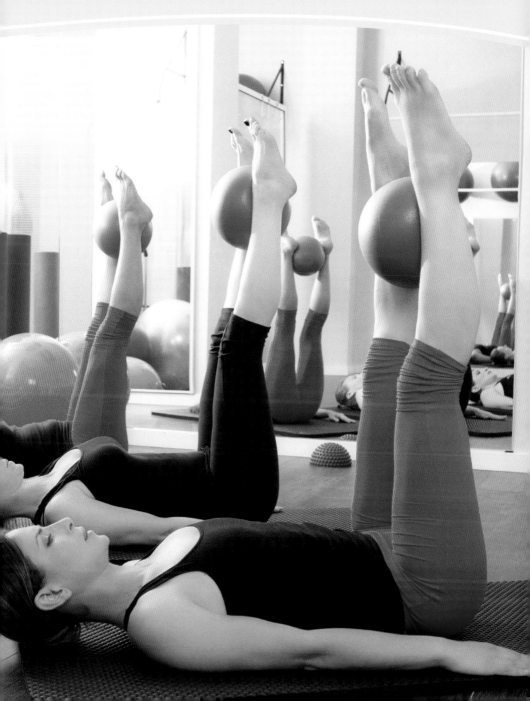

Gym Equipment

Exercising under your own steam is cheap and easy to fit into your schedule, but on a grey day there's a lot to be said for heading to the gym for a cardio workout. You will be able to vary your activities, spending five to ten minutes on different pieces of equipment. Use each machine to the max by testing yourself at different intensity levels, and set targets to increase your speed or distance, with sprints and active rest periods.

Cross-trainer

The cross-trainer, or elliptical, is an excellent choice for a low-impact exercise. It offers aerobic activity that engages your arms and legs, and even your core. The elliptical movement combines the motions used on the bike, stair stepper and treadmill in a smooth, gliding action.

Use the cross-trainer as a gentle warm-up, or push yourself for a more intense workout. Increase the level as high as you can to focus on your legs, or reduce it slightly and engage your arms more, allowing you to step at a higher speed. A person weighing around 10 ½ stone can burn 400 calories in 30 minutes if they work hard on the cross-trainer.

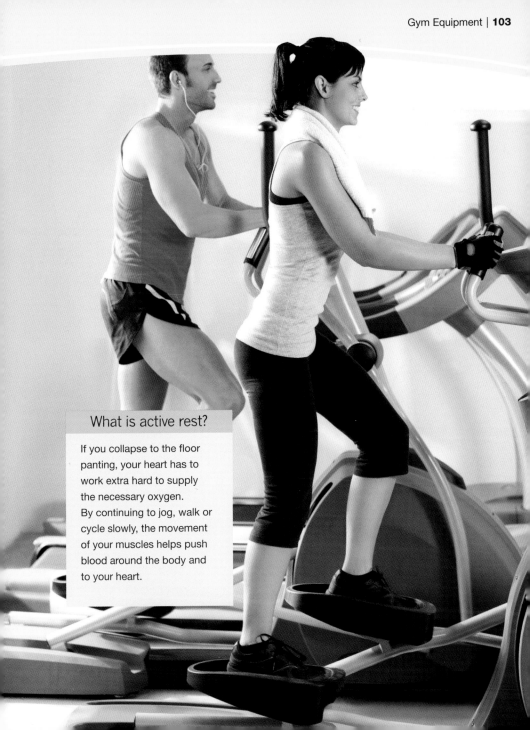

What is active rest?

If you collapse to the floor panting, your heart has to work extra hard to supply the necessary oxygen.
By continuing to jog, walk or cycle slowly, the movement of your muscles helps push blood around the body and to your heart.

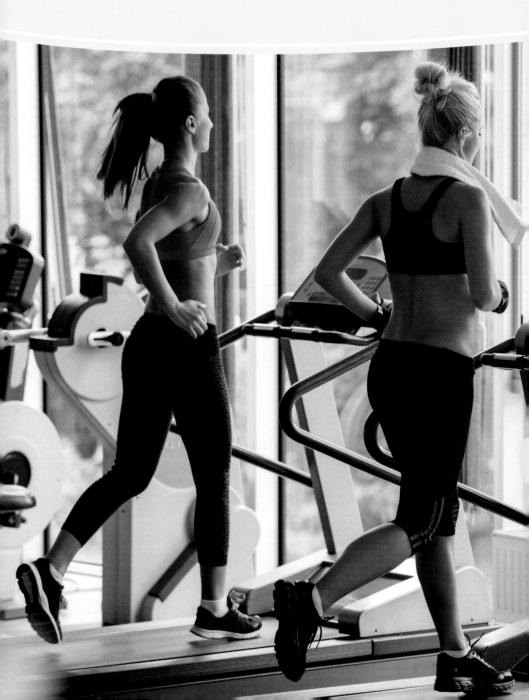

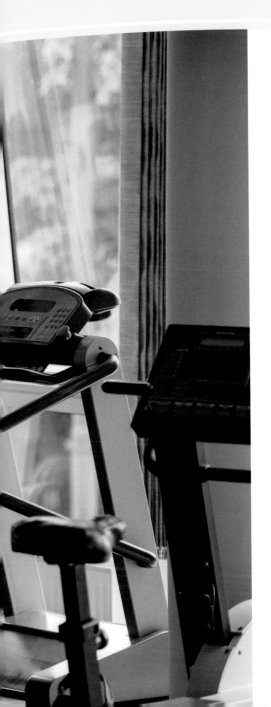

Take to the treadmill

Treadmills are great if it's too icy to risk running outside – or too hot – or you have time to exercise in your lunch break but work in an area that's not conducive to road running. They also offer more shock absorption than you can expect from running outdoors.

Make the most of additional features to get a workout that you wouldn't achieve easily in your locality. Use the incline to run steadily uphill (for an extra burn in your gluteal muscles, to firm your bottom) or choose a setting that varies the hill climbs for you.

Many running machines allow you to track more than just your distance; you can see your pace-per-kilometre and effort level as well. Use the heart rate receiver if it has one to see how efficiently you move from resting rate to high intensity and back again. This allows you to work to your own performance targets, whether it's fat burning or increasing your stamina.

On your bike!

You may find more than one type of
stationary bike in your gym. Recumbent
bikes look as though you are almost lying
down to pedal; they are especially good
for getting your bottom in shape. Upright
bikes work your thighs. Some will have
a digital display to allow you to add hill
climbs or increase the resistance level,
so you have to pedal harder. Spin bikes
feature a small twistable knob to adjust
the resistance; you will usually end up
standing up to pedal at the hardest levels.

Indoor cycling has many benefits, not least
the capacity to go for a ride regardless of
the weather. It offers a safe environment if
you're not confident about cycling in traffic,
and as many hills as you choose, even if
you live in a totally flat area. It also allows
you to exercise your legs without putting
pressure on your joints. The forwards
motion of your legs is kinder to knees than
a running action, and increased strength in
your thigh muscles will protect your knees
from potential injury.

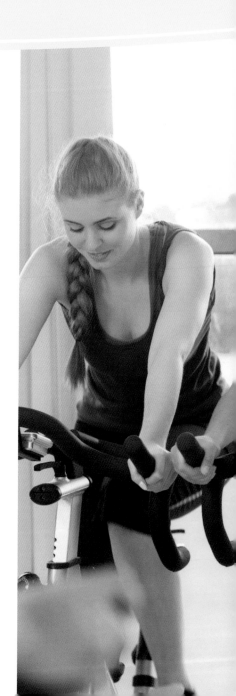

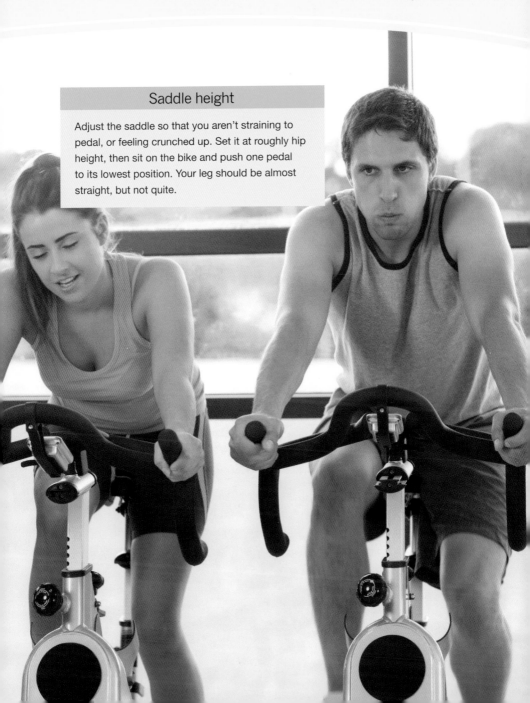

Saddle height

Adjust the saddle so that you aren't straining to pedal, or feeling crunched up. Set it at roughly hip height, then sit on the bike and push one pedal to its lowest position. Your leg should be almost straight, but not quite.

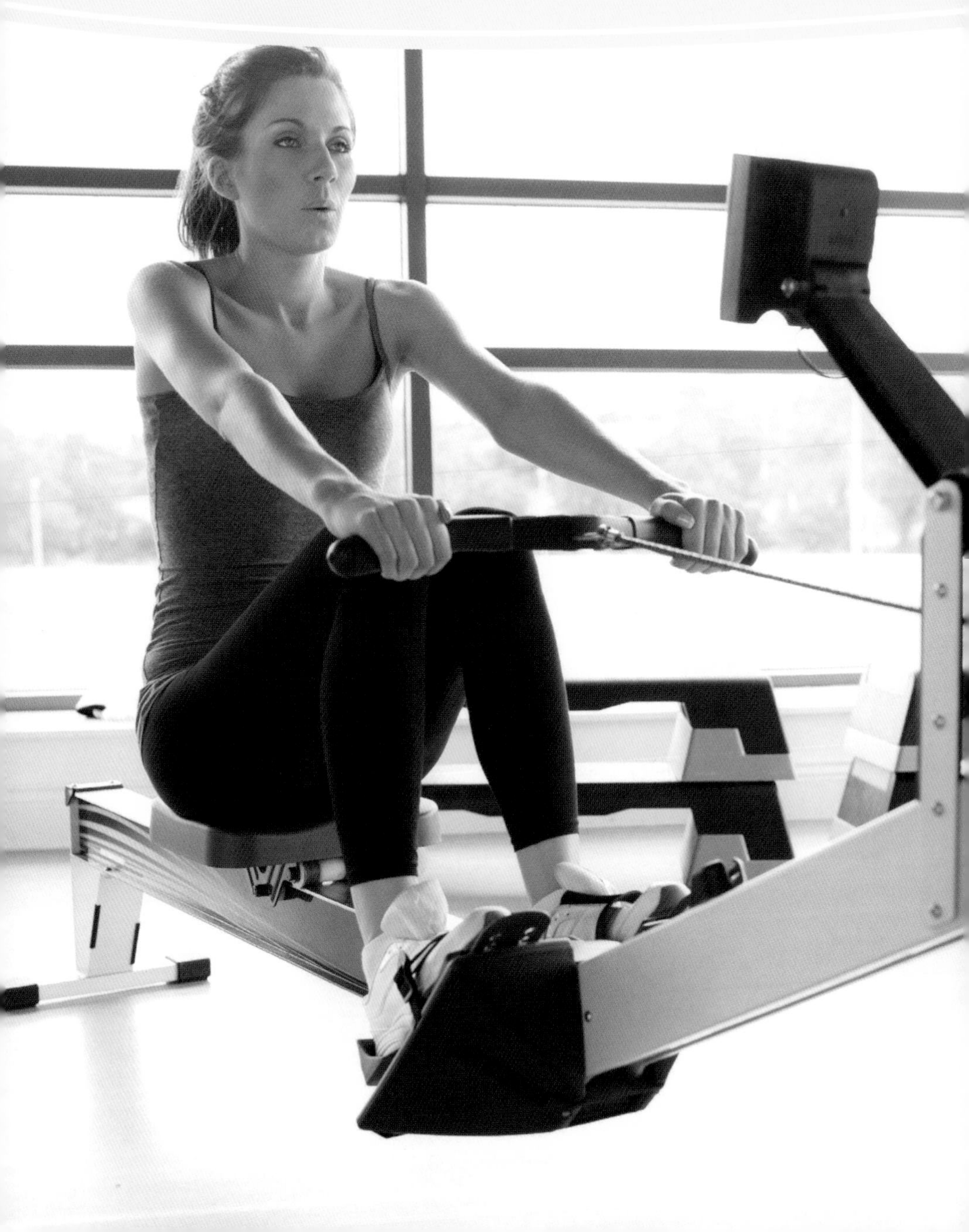

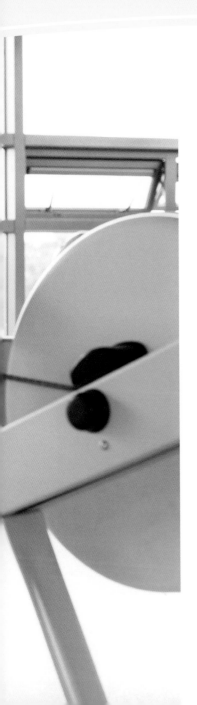

Row your boat

The rowing machine offers an excellent cardio workout that will get your heart pumping hard. Done properly, it engages your leg muscles, stomach and core, arms, shoulders and back. Rowing is great for competitive types; keep a tally of the distance rowed in a set time, and try to beat it, or see how quickly you can reach the 1,000-metre mark, for example.

The basic movement starts with a hard drive through the legs, followed by a strong pull from the arms, and finishes with the torso leaning slightly backwards. The legs pull back in to return to the start position. Row slowly at first and focus on your body to feel how the muscles move, and really engage your thighs, calves and upper body for the maximum effect. Increase your pace to maintain a steady rhythm with strong movements, and push yourself to include sprint intervals for maximum cardio effect.

Super stamina

Rowing can be done in short bursts, to build strength, or longer sessions, to increase stamina and endurance. A 10 ½ stone person should use over 300 calories in 30 minutes.

Weight machines

Bodyweight exercise is the latest buzz-phrase in the fitness world, but don't be afraid to go old-school and give the machines a try. Although they are limited in the range of movement, so you don't use your body in a 'natural', working way, they are good for targeting certain muscles. This can be a benefit if you're working your way back from injury, or want to build strength in a specific part of your body.

Weight machines won't necessarily engage your back, abs and core in the same way that other exercises do, or get you fit for sports. They will, however, allow you to perform actions with your arms and legs that you don't perform so much in daily life. You are most likely to push with your arms, so incorporate more pulling exercises with weights. Add heavier weights to your leg exercises to build strength. The stronger these muscles become, the better able you will be to perform floor exercises, from planks and press-ups to chin-ups and pull-ups.

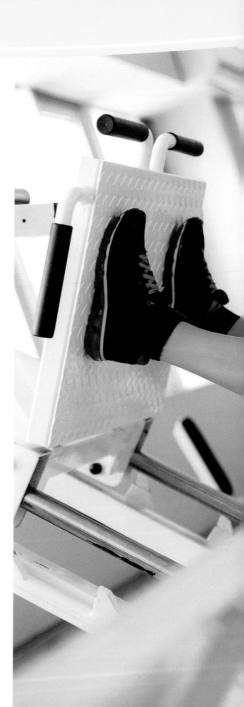

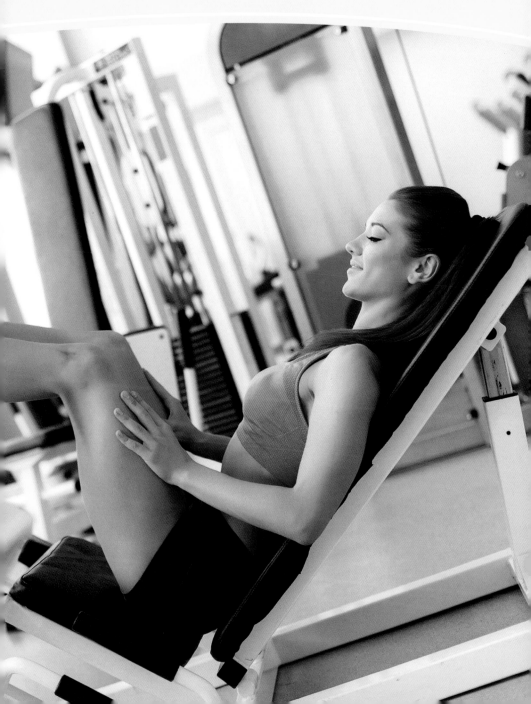

Making Progress

The key to summer fit success is seeing progress. Ultimately, your goal is to look and feel better in your summer clothes, and to enjoy the better weather with a fresh outlook and a fitter lifestyle. Some of these things are unquantifiable; are you happier than you were last summer? How do you measure it? However, many of your goals can be recorded at the beginning of your campaign, and you can keep track of how things are progressing.

Keep a diary, beginning with a note of your starting points: weight, clothes size and your estimation of your own fitness levels. Make a daily note of the things you eat and the exercise you do. Be honest; no one benefits from fibbing about that slice of cheesecake you sneaked in after lunch. However, you will reap rewards from seeing exactly what you need to improve upon.

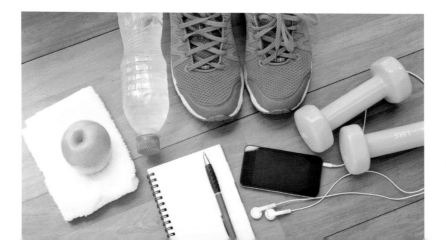

Record and review

Take stock of what you have recorded. Highlight the weak points and aim to replace them with plus points. Feel proud every time you drink camomile tea instead of wine before bed. Smile – inwardly and outwardly – at the extra gym session you squeezed in on Saturday morning. That's what this is all about!

Hopefully, you will soon see improvements in all aspects. Your body will reward your hard work as you get into shape. Not only will you feel and look better in your summer wardrobe, you should have higher energy levels. This in turn will boost you so that you can tackle each day with vigour, and engage in summer activities with zest.

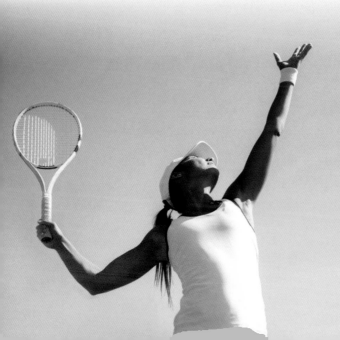

Weighing In

For most people, weight is a good guide to the shape they are in. Take a note of your start weight and keep track of your weight from spring into summer. If you are exercising hard and eating well, you should see your weight fall over the course of a few weeks.

However, don't place too much importance on what the scales say. They are simply a numerical guide to what is happening overall, but not a specific indication of how you are shaping up. Your weight may not change drastically as you burn fat and increase muscle. Muscle is denser than fat, and so your lean, toned body may weigh the same as the softer, squidgier shape you started at – but it will certainly look better in the mirror.

See for yourself

Measuring yourself in other ways can be a better indicator of how your body is changing. Write down your start measurements around your waist, hips, upper arm and upper thigh. Wait a few weeks, and then measure again. Hopefully, as your body becomes firmer, these measurements will reduce slightly. But again, don't rely solely on the numbers, but judge by how you look and feel.

Use your performance as a measure of how much you have achieved. As time passes, you should be running further or faster (or swimming, or cycling), touching your toes more easily, or performing more reps with greater weights. All of these are the best bonus, and something that you will carry forwards into the winter months, even when you start wearing thick jumpers again. Your target now is to avoid hibernation and stay fit far into the next spring, and summer, and beyond. Make a start now with some of the sample workouts on the following pages.

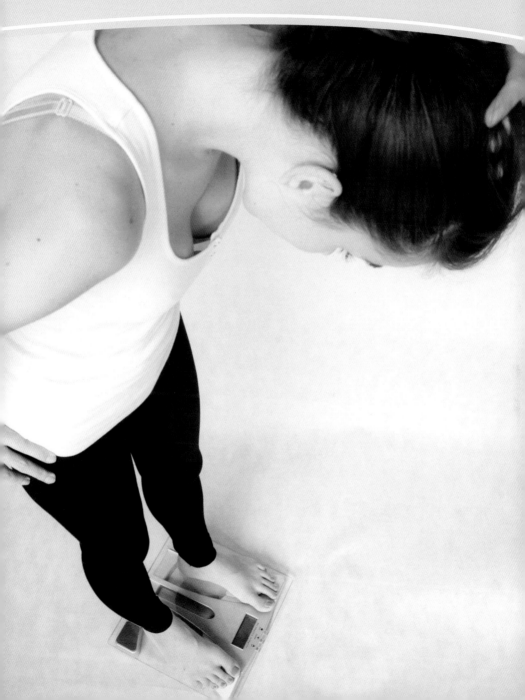

Workouts

10 **Minutes**	If you only have 10 minutes to work out, make it count! You will find all of the exercises in the central section of this book. Don't rest in between; switching exercises will give you a window to bring your breathing under control.
0–2 Minutes	**Squats with bicep curls** – as many reps as you can, without losing form by going too fast. For an extra boost, try pistol squats for the first 30 seconds (no curls).
2–4 Minutes	**Russian twists** – hold a medicine ball or weight in both hands, touching it to the floor each side as you twist.
4–6 Minutes	**Tricep dips** – do in sets of 10, with a 5-second rest between each set.
6–8 Minutes	**Step-up with knee raise** – set as fast a pace as you can to complete as many as possible in the 2 minutes – without stopping
8–10 Minutes	**Bicycle kicks with twist** – touching opposite arm and knee for 1 minute, then rest for 10 seconds, then continue to the end. Don't go too fast as you'll perform them badly. Warm down on the move by stretching out your arms, chest and shoulders, and walking up the stairs with your feet hanging slightly off the back of each step, lowering the heel each time to stretch out the calves.

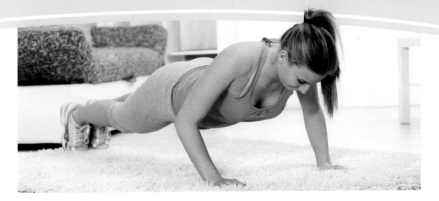

20
Minutes

This is a quick blast workout that will raise your heart rate as well as targeting various muscle groups. It consists of two parts with a 1-minute rest in between. No equipment is required.

Part 1

Perform each of these moves with the number of reps shown, and then repeat until your 10 minutes is up.

a. Mountain climber x 30 (15 on each leg)

b. Squat thrusts x 15

c. Press-ups x 10 (elevated if possible)

d. Side lunge x 20 (10 on each leg)

e. Bird flaps for 30 seconds

Part 2

Rest and drink water, and then start on these moves. Again, repeat until the time is up.

a. Squats x 10

b. Reverse lunge x 20 (10 on each leg)

c. Air circles x 20

d. Superman x 10

e. Plank for 30 seconds

---

30 Minutes

If you have a half-hour window for exercise, use the first part to target your upper and lower body, and finish with 10 minutes of cardio.

Circuits

Perform each of these exercises 10 times, take a drink and then start a new circuit with 10 more reps of each. Stop after 20 minutes.

a. Forward lunge
b. Bridge
c. Press-ups
d. Tricep dips
e. Sit-ups
f. Side plank dip and raise

Cardio

This depends on where you are, but try to alter the intensity. Do 1 minute of average intensity and then up the levels (sprinting or hill climbing) for 30 seconds. You can jog around the park, run up and down the stairs, or choose a machine at the gym. When you're finished, warm down and stretch.

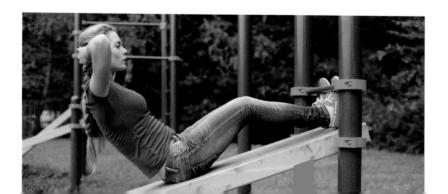

50 **Minutes**	This is ample time for a full workout. Start with a warm up. If you're in the gym, spend 5 minutes on the cross-trainer or your preferred machine. If you're at home jog on the spot.
5–10 Minutes	Start with 30 sit-ups and then do 10 reps each of these three exercises, repeating as many times as possible. Side bends – Double crunches – Dead bug
10–15 Minutes *	**In the gym:** cardio – alternate a steady pace and sprints for 1 minute each. **At home:** alternate step-ups and burpees for 1 minute each.
15–20 Minutes	Do 30 crunches and then 30 seconds each (repeated) of: Wall sit – Lunge walks – Jumping jacks
20–25 Minutes	Repeat * (on a different machine, if possible).
25–30 Minutes	Do 30 punches (with weights, if possible) and then 10 reps each (repeated) of: Tricep dips – Press-ups – Tricep kickbacks
30–35 Minutes	Repeat *
40–45 Minutes	Do 10 reps on each side, repeated, of these: Kneeling leg raise – Donkey kick - Side leg raise
45–50 Minutes	Repeat *, really pushing yourself to the end.

Walking

Walking can just be a stroll in the park – or it can be a power walk that raises your heart rate and tones your legs and bottom. Throw in some arm swings and you will benefit even more. To get an even better bottom-toning boost, squeeze your glutes during your walk.

You can adjust your stride during your walk to focus the work on different muscle groups. Grab a friend and get going – the following workout is best done with someone else so you don't feel self-conscious.

Begin with a 5-minute walk at a comfortable (not slow) pace to warm up. Now speed up, taking longer strides than normal. Walk like this at 1-minute intervals with a comfortable pace, for 5 minutes. Next, alternate 1-minute intervals of lunge-walking with a moderately paced walk. Sink low into the lunge to really work your legs and bottom. Repeat these two sequences for the duration of your walk, with a 5-minute stroll at the end to cool down.

Aim to walk for 30 minutes, if possible. That's plenty of time to catch up on all the chat!

Running

Whether you're a beginner or a more experienced runner, you can always benefit from interval training. The idea is to speed up and slow down during your running time. It has many plus points: it helps trim your tummy and waist, increases your metabolism during rest, and burns more calories in the time you devote to training. On your marks, get set, go!

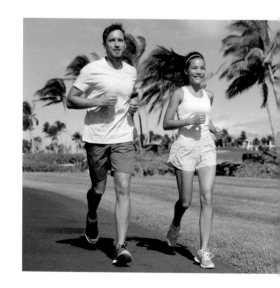

Intermediate running intervals

This workout is aimed at runners with limited experience. If you are new to running, or training for an event, check the adjustments beneath the workout.

0–5 Minutes	Warm up (run at a slow but steady pace).
5–7.5 Minutes	Speed up to a sprint.
7.5–10 Minutes	Slow down to a medium pace where running is comfortable but not slow.
10–12.5 Minutes	Speed up to a faster pace than your first sprint.
12.5–15 Minutes	Return to medium pace.
15–17.5 Minutes	Sprint as fast as you can.
17.5–20 Minutes	Return to medium pace.

To cool down, slow down for 5 more minutes. Spend a few minutes stretching out your legs when you're done.

Beginner level

Reduce the sprint time to 1 minute, or set a distance target – for example, to the end of the road.

Advanced level

Speed up your sprints, run faster than a medium pace during the rest periods, and gradually reduce the rest periods to 30 seconds or a minute.

Swimming

It's easy to drift through endless lengths of the pool without really concentrating on what you are trying to achieve – improved fitness with toned legs and arms. Take a tip from endurance athletes and devise a workout before you dive in.

Begin with backstroke to warm up your muscles, stretch out your shoulders and gently raise your heart rate.

For endurance, do sets of laps at the fastest sprint speed (freestyle or front crawl) that you can manage:

8 lengths then active rest (breaststroke for 2 lengths)

4 lengths then active rest

2 lengths then active rest

1 length then switch onto your back

Of course, if you're already a strong swimmer, you should repeat this sequence to add extra distance.

For toned legs, swim 2 lengths holding a float in front of you to focus the work onto your lower body.

Use your last 5 minutes in the pool to cool down, decrease your heart rate, and to avoid the build up of lactic acid in your muscles. Swim a slow crawl, back and front, and extend your arms to the max to stretch out your muscles.

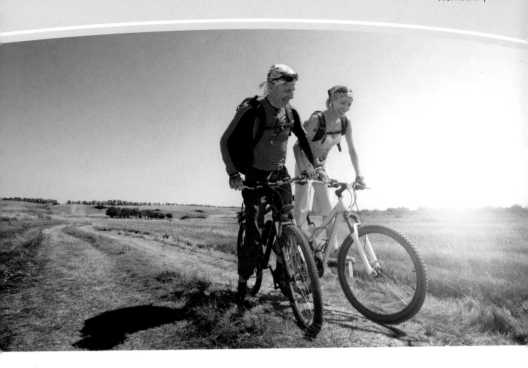

Cycling

Interval training isn't only for runners. Cyclists will also benefit from pushing themselves hard and fast for short spells. As well as the increased fat burning and raised metabolic rate, you will get fit in a shorter space of time, saving yourself hours of pootling around the countryside and getting saddle sore.

Ease yourself into your ride (whether it's outdoors or on a stationary bike) with a 5-minute warm-up at a slow to steady pace.

Now spend the next 9 minutes doing intervals. Pedal hard and fast for just 30 seconds, and then drop back to a medium pace (where you could carry out a conversation but are still working reasonably hard) for 1 minute. You will fit six bursts of speed and rest into this time. Warm down for 5 more minutes at a steady pace.

As your fitness improves, add more intervals, or reduce the rest time to 30 seconds.

Reap the Rewards

It's easy to make a start on a fitness campaign, but it's an awful lot harder to stick with it. Those who have the greatest success are the ones who take on board the permanence of the changes they are making, rather than looking for a quick fix.

When you reach the tricky weeks after the 'honeymoon period' is over, you may need to incentivise yourself. Reward yourself with non-food treats that allow you to enjoy the new you. Have a massage on your aching – but newly toned – muscles. Buy a new nail varnish and paint your toenails to show off at the pool. Accept that you're on a long journey, and that you will need to work for a good few months before your new regime becomes a habit that carries you through the hard times.

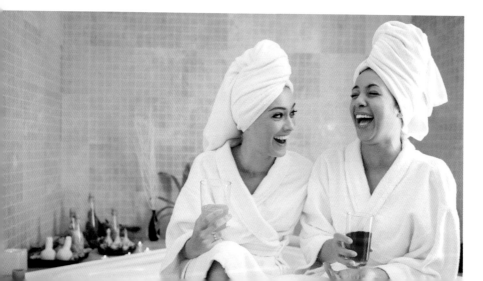

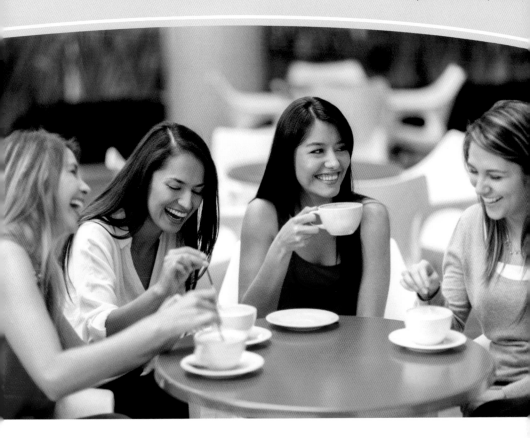

Rest and relax

Take time off, too. Allow yourself the luxury of taking a gentle walk and enjoying nature, instead of feeling the burn as you race along. Meet up with friends and bask in the compliments about how great you look. Chances are that you will have a new glow about you if you are really feeling great about yourself.

Don't forget, your body needs time to recover after you've worked it hard. Sleep and rest are vital for well-being. Studies show that the recommended 150 minutes of exercise each week can improve sleep quality by up to 65 per cent and reduce the feeling of tiredness during the day. In addition, your newly boosted metabolism is still working overtime while you slumber. Sweet dreams, indeed!

Abs: the abdominal muscles of the stomach and waist: the rectus and transversus abdominis and external and internal obliques, which move and support your spine and upper body.

Barbell: a metal bar with interchangeable weights attached at each end.

Bone density: a measurement of the amount of minerals (including calcium) in a volume of bone; used to determine bone strength and vulnerability to fractures and osteoporosis.

Core strength: the strength of the collective muscles of the torso, which help to keep the body stable and balanced during motion and rest.

Dumbbell: a short bar with weights at each end, often used in pairs. The weights may be fixed or interchangeable.

Exercise ball: a large inflatable ball used to offer resistance or support during exercise; also called a Swiss ball, body ball, yoga ball or gym ball.

Fibre: found in plant-based foods, fibre is not absorbed by the body so offers no nutrients, but helps the body process food, lowers blood cholesterol, and helps you to feel full after eating.

Flexed feet: with the toes pulled towards the body instead of pointed away from the body.

Glutes: any of the three large muscles in the buttock that move the thigh and hip.

High/low impact: high impact movements involve more direct force on the body than low impact movements, usually because of jumping and landing on hard ground.

Kettlebell: a spherical weight with a single handle over the top.

Medicine ball: an extremely heavy ball, roughly the size of a basketball, used for strength training.

Obliques: the muscles at the sides of the torso: external and internal, which cross diagonally from beneath your ribs to your pelvis; they help you twist and bend at the waist.

Protein: gained from animal sources (meat and dairy) and seeds and legumes, protein helps to build, replace and maintain body tissue such as muscle and red blood cells.

Quads: a large muscle group at the front of the thigh, containing four muscles which support and extend (straighten) the knee in opposition to the hamstring and gluteal muscles.

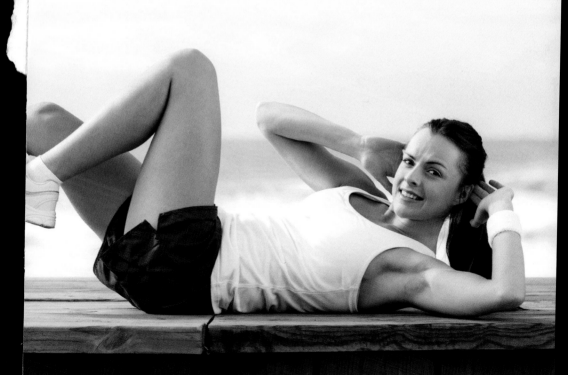

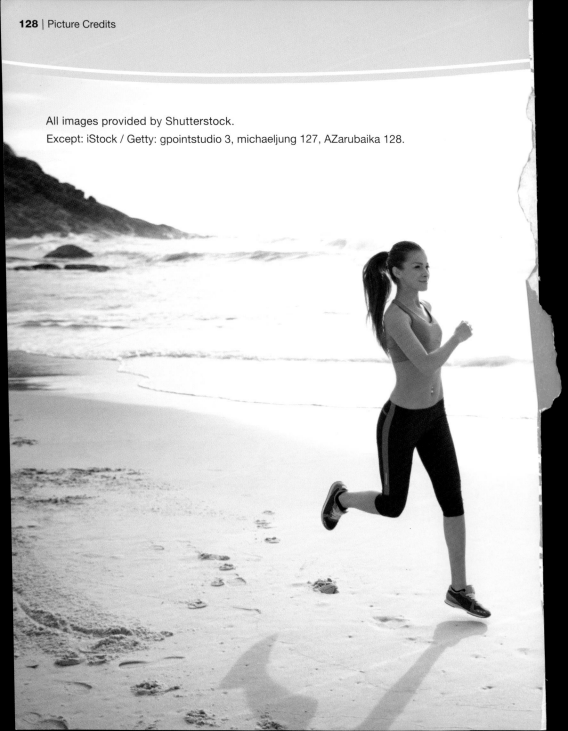